Treating Fearful Dental Patients

A PATIENT MANAGEMENT HANDBOOK

Second Edition, Revised

Treating Fearful Dental Patients

A PATIENT MANAGEMENT HANDBOOK

Second Edition, Revised

Peter Milgrom, D.D.S.
Professor, Department of Dental Public Health Sciences
University of Washington School of Dentistry
Seattle, Washington

Philip Weinstein, Ph.D.
Professor, Department of Dental Public Health Sciences
University of Washington School of Dentistry
Seattle, Washington

Tracy Getz, M.S.
Lecturer, Department of Dental Public Health Sciences
University of Washington School of Dentistry
Seattle, Washington

**University of Washington
Continuing Dental Education**

Library of Congress Cataloging in Publication Data

Main entry under title:

Treating fearful dental patients.

    Bibliography: p.
    1. Dentistry—Psychological aspects. 2. Fear. 3. Dentist and patient.
I. Milgrom, Peter. [DNLM: 1. Fear. 2. Patients—psychology. 3. Dental
Care—psychology. 4. Dentist-Patient Relations.   WU 61 T784]
RK53.T74 (1985) 1995   617.6′0019 84-23726
ISBN 1-880291-01-0

© 1995 by Continuing Dental Education
University of Washington, Seattle, Washington 98195
(206) 543-5444

10 9 8 7 6 5 4 3 2 1

Printed in the United States of America

CONTENTS

FOREWORD

This book is a treatise about managing fearful dental patients and, to a more limited extent, dealing with other behavioral problems which also interfere with dental treatment. As we shall see, its mission is much broader than this statement would indicate.

The history of dental fears predates modern dentistry. Some five centuries ago, Albrecht Dürer produced engravings showing extreme patient reactions to exodontia. One can find examples today in cartoons where fear reactions to dental treatment are illustrated. Although some practitioners take offense at such cartoons, these illustrations allow us to draw two important conclusions. First, dental fears are widely found in the population. As the reader will find, this conclusion is also supported by population surveys. Second, dental fears are *socially acceptable*. Most fear behaviors are *not* socially acceptable. The fact that dental fears are so widespread may account for this phenomenon. This social acceptability makes it easier for patients to rationalize their fear behavior. It makes it easier to develop and maintain the fear. It also makes the job of the clinician more difficult in any attempt to overcome the fear so that treatment may be facilitated.

The development of a body of knowledge concerning what we now refer to as "Behavioral Science in Dentistry" is fairly recent. Until the late 1950s most discussions of dental fear and behavioral management were tied to psychoanalytic or Freudian theory. It may have been enlightening for some practitioners to learn than dental procedures such as exodontia aroused castration anxiety, but this knowledge was of little help in developing management techniques. More behaviorally oriented articles began to appear in dental journals at the same time as the federal government began pumping money into the health education system because of a perceived shortage of physicians and dentists. This infusion of new money into the health care system and the increased demand for knowledge of patient management techniques combined to provide the impetus for the development of behavioral sciences in both medicine and dentistry. By 1960, the *Zeitgeist* was right for the explosive emergence of behavioral science in dental education.

Three broad areas of behavioral issues in dentistry began to be addressed. These areas included social and personality factors in utilization of dental services; issues related to the characteristics of dental students and educational variables in training; and finally, approaches to the assessment and management of dental anxiety or fear in patients. One of the first of the new behavioral scientists was Steve Kegeles, a social psychologist, who was hired by the U.S. Public Health Service in the late 1950s. He conducted studies of water fluoridation, factors related to acceptance of dental care, and factors related to seeking care. Subsequently, Bob O'Shea and, eventually, Lois Cohen (both of them sociologists) were also hired by the P.H.S. Division of Dental Health. They continued the investigations of factors associated with patient acceptance of treatment as well as issues related to training and continuing education of dentists.

While this trend had begun in the late 1950s in Washington, D.C., another was beginning elsewhere. A Canadian dentist named Grant Phipps had tired of running a successful practice and returned to college where he "discovered" psychology. He received his Ph.D. in clinical psychology in 1960 and went to the University of Pittsburgh and established the first Department of Behavioral Science in a dental school. He obtained an National Institutes of Health (N.I.H.) training grant to educate psychology researchers in problems relevant to dentistry. His first graduate was Dick Mackenzie—a dentist—who received his doctorate in psychology. Mackenzie succeeded Phipps as chair of the department and developed what was then the most extensive behavioral science curriculum in a dental school. His major focus was on educational issues in dental training. He eventually went on to chair the department at the University of Florida.

Phipps went to Buffalo in 1964 where he established another Department of Behavioral Science and received another training grant. At Buffalo, he hired me, Elliot Gale and Bob O'Shea. I began to investigate general issues related to dental anxiety including assessment. Gale focused on patient treatment from the beginning and published a number of papers on treatment of phobic patients and issues related to that treatment. O'Shea was involved in a seminal study of Medicaid utilization. Every training program has a star and ours is Bill Ayer who now holds an endowed chair at Northwestern University School of Dentistry.

There were a number of other contributors to behavioral science during the 1960s. Don Giddon, a dentist and psychologist from Harvard, is probably best known during this period for his research on personality factors associated with acute necrotizing ulcerative gingivitis. Sandy Rosenzweig at Tufts conducted research on stress factors in the etiology of cleft palate. Ernie Clark, also at Tufts, developed a rigorous and well-conceptualized research program in psychosomatics. Dick Evans, a psychologist at the University of Houston, also had a training grant, published a number of papers on the impact of behavioral science on dentistry, and investigated fear arousal and persuasion on changes in oral hygiene behavior. Aaron Katcher, a psychiatrist at the University of Pennsylvania, was chair of Behavioral Science in Dentistry and conducted research on behavioral variables in illness.

Another psychiatrist, Bud Baldwin, conducted research on personality factors in orthodontic treatment and extractions in children. He became chair of the new department at the University of Connecticut School of Dentistry with an outstanding group of faculty: Steve Kegeles, Matt Weisenberg, and Howard Bailit. In New York City, Sam Dworkin did a doctoral dissertation in psychology which demonstrated that a dental context made people perceive pain much more readily than a non-dental context. He also began to study student performance on the Dental Aptitude Test and spearheaded efforts to put behavioral science material on the National Board examinations.

It is interesting to note that almost all of this activity in dental behavioral sciences occurred in the eastern United States and then seemed to move west. One exception to this was Tim Smith who brought behavioral science to Kentucky during this period. Another exception was Larry Meskin at the University of Minnesota who hired Mike Loupe and did studies of dental manpower issues during the 1960s.

It was during the middle 1960s that we felt it would be desirable for the people in dental behavioral science to associate more closely with each other and attempt to find our own niche in the principal professional research and teaching organizations. Elliot Gale and I invited every behavioral person we could find at the 1967 meeting of the International Association for Dental Research to meet with us to discuss the limited goal of getting our own place on the annual program. Shortly thereafter, Lois Cohen called a meeting of department chairs and program directors to establish the Behavioral Scientists in Dental Research organization. Grant Phipps was the first president. This organization became the Behavioral Science Group of IADR and also affiliated with the Federation Dentaire Internationale. Thus, within a decade, dental behavioral science had rapidly evolved with many people conducting research on a variety of issues and had formed its own professional interest group.

The decade of the 1970s was an era of expansion and consolidation so that nearly every American dental school had some behavioral science representation included in its faculty and curriculum. The development which was occurring was very important for dental curricula. What had once began as "junior" psychology or psychiatry courses for dental students were now becoming applied dental behavioral courses based on research conducted in behavioral science and/or community dentistry. The authors of this book were part of the expansion occurring during this period and developed one of the most important and productive research groups in dental behavioral science.

It was also during the 1970s that behavioral science "burst forth" in dental schools on the international scene. Research and curriculum development occurred in England, Ireland, the Scandinavian countries, Netherlands, Japan, and, most recently, Israel. This broad based development led to an extensive accumulation of applied knowledge which continued to be supplemented through the 1980s and into the 1990s.

Probably, the most important development during the 1980s was the advent of dental fear clinics. Groups of psychologists and dentists established clinical facilities for treating fearful patients and for training dentists to manage such patients. It is not easy to establish a fear clinic. It is not a matter of hanging out a shingle and finding patients at the door ready to be treated. The patients only want to come when they are in distress—and often, not even then. A fearful patient may learn of the existence of a clinic and, finally, a year or two later come for treatment. Eventually, a clinic becomes solidly established. The clinic at the University of Washington has been in operation for over a decade and has become an important treatment and training facility.

The problem of patient fear in the dental office, as we have noted, is an age old phenomenon. One might well wonder how people can develop such counter-productive fear behaviors. The authors have provided an excellent discussion of the various ways fear can develop. I must caution the reader, however, that in any given case, it is nearly impossible to discover the original source of the patient's fear. No matter how "socially acceptable" dental fear may be, it is still irrational behavior. People who engage in irrational behavior give themselves reasons for their behavior. They attempt to provide a rational basis for the fear. Usually, there is no way to determine how veridical the patient's explanation may be. Fortunately, it doesn't matter! The patient may be "treated" or managed without reference to the original cause of the fear.

This book is mostly about managing fearful dental patients. What one finds in reading it is a combination of sound psychological principles and compassionate common sense. After three decades of association with dental behavioral science, I have come to the conclusion that what is presented in this book is not merely useful material for managing fearful patients but a general approach which should be used with all patients. I would recommend that it be read with that proviso in mind.

Norman L. Corah, Ph.D.
Professor of Behavioral Science
School of Dental Medicine
State University of New York at Buffalo

DEDICATION

This edition of our text is dedicated to the devoted and hardworking staff of the Dental Fears Research Clinic at the University of Washington. Treating fearful patients all day long requires a team effort, a high level of interpersonal skill, and a considerable amount of patience, perseverance, and faith. We openly acknowledge that we could not be successful without the following members of our team: Kathy Schaefer, our dental assistant; our dental hygienists, Marilynn Rothen and Agnes Spadafora; our patient services coordinator, Coral Namisnak; and our billing representative, Colleen King.

We would like to express our sincere gratitude to the Office Staff of our department whose support was crucial to the success of this project and, especially, to Alison Ayers-Maynard for her capable word-processing skills, and to Reinhard "Ron" Hahn who created the camera-ready manuscript. Finally, we would like to thank our editor, Connie Pious, for her expertise with the written word and her dedication to detail.

Peter Milgrom
Philip Weinstein
Tracy Getz

INTRODUCTION TO THE SECOND EDITION

Treating Fearful Dental Patients, initially conceived in 1984 and published in 1985, was the first textbook specifically written for dental personnel and students on the management of the fearful and phobic dental patient. It brought together for the first time knowledge and expertise from the field of psychology on the treatment of anxiety disorders and applied it to the problems that dental personnel all too commonly face with patients. Now, with an additional 10 years of work with fearful patients we are pleased to present this second edition. It is a result of our direct clinical work with patients in the Dental Fears Research Clinic at the University of Washington, innumerable consultations and conversations with colleagues worldwide and, finally, the research findings of our own and others' work with this population.

When we first began seeing only fearful patients in 1982 we were one of two such clinics worldwide. Today, we know of fifteen such clinics associated with hospitals or dental schools, and the number continues to grow. The dental profession has come to recognize both the extent of the problem, and that there are specific strategies which practitioners can employ to successfully treat fearful patients.

In this text we have attempted to bring together the best of the most recent research findings with our clinical experience managing fearful patients. We blend results from our research in this area with clinical insights to illustrate and enhance the usefulness of each. We have purposely attempted to walk the thin line between a scholarly presentation and an anecdotal approach to create a readable, useful, but scientific text.

This book was conceived as a practical handbook for both students and practicing professionals, dentists, dental hygienists, and assistants. We will begin with a model for understanding the etiology and treatment of fear. We will then discuss diagnosis, and examine common patterns (or clusters) of patient dental fears. Finally, we will teach you how to use diagnostic information to select appropriate treatments from a wide range of practical pharmacological and psychological strategies to most effectively address the specific concerns of a particular patient.

Why learn "special" skills to treat the fearful patient?

There are three very apparent reasons. The first involves the issue of "busyness." Studies indicate that only about one half of the American population goes to the dentist once a year. Studies have also shown that somewhere between six percent and 14 percent of the American population (14,000,000–34,000,000) avoid dentistry completely because of fear. It is estimated that another 20–30 percent dislike dentistry enough to be only occasional users. Fear is a very real barrier to seeking dental services and should be dealt with. In addition, if you reduce an individual's anxiety, you increase the probability that he will follow through on recommended treatment and will return for recall. We believe that the ability to recognize and successfully treat the anxious patient results in many new patients who will stay the course and fewer fear-related cancellations and failures.

Secondly, learning to treat the fearful patient will reduce your own personal stress level. Surveys have repeatedly shown that the most frustrating aspect of dental practice is working with the "difficult" patient. By learning skills to help you work with the fearful patient, you will reduce the stress of dental practice and the possibility of professional burnout.

Finally, there is the personal reward of helping a person overcome a difficult barrier. Long after we forget our finest technical accomplishments, we have found that we remember and take satisfaction from having been able to truly make a significant difference in another person's life.

Financial considerations in the treatment of fearful patients

One frequently asked question is, "How can I afford to spend 'extra' time with a fearful patient helping him feel more comfortable? I have a business to run." Our answer to that is another question. When was the last time you saw a patient needing 2,000 to 4,000 dollars worth of dental care who would describe going to the dentist as an easy experience? Most big cases result from years of neglect, and the patients who most need our services are the very people who are least tolerant of dental treatment. It has been our experience that the "extra" time and effort required to reduce a patient's fears to a manageable level are initial investments which pay long-term personal, professional, and financial dividends.

However, we do not believe that the time spent working with patients to help them tolerate treatment more comfortably should simply be considered the price of doing business, or that it ought to be "given" away. The skills that you will learn in this book are valuable, and there are definite costs to you in delivering them. We believe that it is legitimate to charge a patient for a well thought out and planned "fear reduction" program. There are several factors to consider in thinking about how to charge a patient. First, who in your office will actually do the work? Consider a patient who has a severe gagging problem and can not tolerate the x-rays or impressions needed for crown and bridge work. The best person in the office to work on desensitizing the patient (see Chapter 8) may be your dental assistant. For her services you may decide to charge only a nominal fee for the one to three hours which may be required. On the other hand, if the patient is extremely needle phobic (see Chapter 8) and hygienists in your state can not give injections, the patient may have to be charged a few hundred dollars for the dentist's time. Some practitioners make such fees "refundable" if the patient successfully follows through with treatment. For example, if the patient completes his endodontic work and the bridge construction, the initial fee for the needle desensitization is applied against the co-payment due on the work. Thus, the patient is given an incentive to complete treatment and his resistance to "practice sessions" is lowered. Other patients simply need a lesson or two in how to cope more effectively with their fears, and a flat fee may be the simplest and most expedient method of handling this treatment.

Another way of looking at the cost of extra time spent is to ask yourself, "What is the cost of a patient not showing up for a scheduled crown preparation, or canceling at the last minute?" Patients who "chicken out" are very costly. If you can learn to diagnose these problems and address them directly to help the patient work through her fears, you could *give away* that "extra" time and find your practice both less frustrating and more financially rewarding.

About the Dental Fears Research Clinic

The Clinic operates as a full fee-for-service faculty practice within the School of Dentistry at the University of Washington in Seattle, Washington. The overhead is comparable to that of an independent practice. Although we do treat difficult children, the primary mission of the clinic is to work with fearful adults. Currently, the average age of our patients is 38. Sixty five percent are female. The average time since a new patient of our clinic has last seen a dentist is 6.8 years, ranging from one day to 36 years. While we, like most practitioners, take some "low-fee" patients, the vast majority of our patients are employed and insured.

READER FEEDBACK FORM

We have found the techniques and procedures described in this book to be helpful to our patients and have tried to convey these and the current research in fear treatment to you. However, we realize that there may be omissions and that we may not have the answers for every patient in your practice. We may not have described our techniques in a way that allowed you to directly apply them to your patients.

To help us make future editions of this book more useful to the provider, we would greatly appreciate your responses to the questions below. Please tell us what features and areas of this book you found useful and those which were not helpful or useful, and address your reponses to:

Dr. Peter Milgrom
University of Washington
Dental Fears Research Clinic
Box 357475
Seattle, Washington 98195-7475
FAX: (206) 685-4258

1. Please describe those features of the book that you found most useful in understanding and treating fearful patients.

_____

_____

_____

_____

2. Note those features or areas of the book that were not useful, were confusing, or that did not seem to work for you.

_____

_____

_____

_____

3. Describe any specific changes you think will enhance the book's clinical usefulness.

_____

_____

_____

4. Describe any cases in which you were able to successfully apply the procedures described to reduce a patient's fears. Please include patient characteristics and the procedures you used.

_____

_____

_____

5. Describe any cases in which you were unable to apply these techniques. Where and how did the book fail to give you what was needed? Please give patient details and what you tried that did not seem to work.

_____

_____

_____

6. Any other comments?

_____

_____

_____

7. Your name and address: (optional)

_____

_____

_____

ONE

The Problem of
Fear in Dentistry

Joan is a 36-year-old, college educated mother of two children. Joan had avoided dentistry totally for the past six years. Not only did she not go herself, she could not even take her children to the pediatric dentist. At her husband's urging, she finally consented to go for an examination, but only if he made the appointment. Even though she was given nitrous oxide, Joan had an intense fear reaction during the examination. Within minutes she was virtually soaked with perspiration and experienced shortness of breath, muscle tension, weakness in her knees, and nausea. She felt an overpowering desire to get out of the office, which she did with the examination only partially completed. Afterwards, she felt "humiliated, embarrassed, and childish. My children can be braver than I was."

Intense fear is one of the most debilitating and agonizing human emotional experiences. It is also one of the most necessary and adaptive emotions. Fear is the motivating force that keeps us from dangers. Although the capacity to experience fear is an innate biological function, our responses of fear to certain objects and situations are largely acquired through our daily learning experiences. As children, we are taught that it is dangerous to play with fire, to play in the street, to talk to strangers, or to venture too far from home. Indeed, a large part of our early learning consists of learning to identify and to avoid potential threats to our well-being.

The development of fear responses to potentially threatening situations is normal, natural, and adaptive. However, acquiring fear responses to perceived threats can proceed in a seemingly non-rational and indiscriminant manner. That is, fear can become associated with a wide variety of environmental objects and situations. Some may pose actual serious threats and the fear response therefore appears "rational." Other fear responses may be clearly "irrational," while yet others may have some degree of rationality but appear out of proportion to the actual threat.

However, it is important to realize that what determines a person's reaction to a situation is not an outsider's view or judgment of the actual or potential threat. It is a result of the individual's own personal perception of the situation, based on his past experiences and interpretation of the present situation.

Joan's earliest memory of dentistry was of the time when she accompanied her mother to the dentist: "I remember waiting in the car. I could see my mother in the chair through a window. She was crying and the dentist was scolding her. I saw the dentist place a cloth over mother's head and face and leave the room. When mother returned to the car she was still crying and very upset."

A powerful and frightening message had been communicated to Joan: "The dentist hurt my mother and he could also hurt me." When Joan was later taken to this same dentist, he scolded her for being a "brat." Out of what she felt was self-defense, she bit his finger when he tried to examine her teeth. Later, she recalled a number of subsequent appointments with this dentist, all of which were reported to be very frightening and painful. These experiences fulfilled her negative expectations concerning dentistry which began with her earlier observation of her mother's experience.

This history of Joan's reactions and early experiences with dentistry is not uncommon among fearful patients. Although briefly described, it illustrates several points concerning dental fear which we will make repeatedly and describe in greater detail throughout this book. First, in all other aspects of her life, Joan was an intelligent, stable, and responsible person. She was a good mother to her children, a good wife to her husband; she maintained her household and a small farm; and she had no other problems requiring psychological intervention. Her reaction to dentistry was the only area of her life she was unable to cope with. This is true of most fearful patients. Second, her seemingly irrational reaction, as viewed from the outside, becomes more understandable and "rational" after we consider her early experiences and associations with dentists. From her experiences, she perceived dentistry as a threat to her well-being. The fear kept her from re-experiencing dentistry, an event that could have changed this perception. Further, if an assessment of her previous dental experiences had been conducted, she would have been spared the trauma and humiliation she experienced. Treatment for her fear could have begun sooner.

Joan was referred to our clinic. We were able to help her overcome her fear of dentistry in a very short time by applying the assessment and treatment procedures described in this book. Because she had avoided treatment for so long, she needed extensive restorative treatment. Within the two months following treatment for her fear, she made and kept five treatment appointments. Further, she felt proud of herself for having conquered her fear, for getting the needed dental treatment, and for finally being able to take her children to the pediatric dentist. This treatment was effective because a program was designed for her specific needs and allowed her to be carefully re-introduced to dentistry by a skillful and concerned dentist.

DEFINITIONS OF FEAR TERMINOLOGY

Thus far we have used the term *fear* without providing a definition. Although most people intuitively know what fear is, it is important to clarify more precisely what we mean by it, and how it differs from the related terms of *anxiety* and *phobia*.

Fear

Fear is an individual's emotional response to a perceived threat or danger. This response is composed of three related components: (1) an unpleasant cognitive state, such as the feeling that something terrible is going to happen; (2) physiologic changes, primarily involving activation of the sympathetic branch of the autonomic nervous system (intense fear reactions will typically include tachycardia, profuse perspiration, respiration changes such as hyperventilation, muscle tension, gastrointestinal upset, and other physiologic signs of emotional arousal); and (3) overt behavioral movements, such as jitteriness, shakes, pacing, and attempts to escape or avoid the perceived threat.

This constellation of fear responses is called the "fight or flight" response (Cannon, 1929). The arousal of fear is seen as generally adaptive because it prepares and mobilizes the body to confront (fight) the threat or to escape from it (flight). We will discuss this fear response and its components in greater detail in Chapter 3.

Anxiety

Anxiety is frequently used to denote an emotional experience similar to fear as we have defined it. In fact, there are some writers who use the two terms synonymously. However, we find it useful to differentiate between the two while recognizing that the responses are similar. We use the term anxiety to denote responses to situations in which the source of threat to the individual is ill-defined, ambiguous, or not immediately present. In other words, anxiety is used to denote reactions to non-immediate situations. For example, one who reacts emotionally to the anticipation of some *future* event would be said to experience "anticipatory anxiety." Accordingly, a person confronting a mugger on a dark street, who experiences apprehension and increased heart rate and feels like running, would be said to be *fearful*. On the other hand, a person who, in the safety of his own home, senses a feeling of dread, whose heart races, and who begins to shake all over at the thought that next week he may confront a mugger would be experiencing anxiety. The major difference is the immediacy of the stimulus.

Phobia

Yet another term used to denote these same responses is phobia. Phobia is a special form of intense fear. The *Diagnostic and Statistical Manual* (DSM IV, 1994) of the American Psychiatric Association defines phobia as a "... marked and persistent fear of clearly discernable, circumscribed objects or situations. Exposure to the phobic stimulus almost invariably provokes an immediate anxiety response" (APA, 1994, p. 405).

This statement goes on to note that when the avoidance is of such proportion that it causes significant distress or interferes with one's social or role functioning, the reaction qualifies as a phobia.

Other characterizations of phobias include statements that they cannot be explained or reasoned away and that they are beyond voluntary control (Marks, 1969). According to these criteria, Joan's reaction to having a dental exam would clearly qualify for the diagnosis of phobia.

As we will see, reactions to dentistry can come in all degrees of intensity and rationality. That is, some people have only mild apprehension, which causes little problem, while others may avoid even the thought or word "dentistry" at all cost.

AN APPROACH-AVOIDANCE CONCEPTUALIZATION FOR DETERMINING THE DEGREE OF PATIENT FEAR

In this section we describe a patient classification system that we have found useful in treatment. It is based in part on the concepts of approach and avoidance tendencies originally described by Lewin (1931) and later explicated by Dollard and Miller (1950) from their research on the nature and effects of fear. Before describing the classifications, we will outline the concepts of the *approach-avoidance conflict.*

An approach-avoidance conflict exists when a person has two competing tendencies with respect to a single situation. That is, a person may want to attain a goal but at the same time avoid it. Relating this to dentistry, we can envision a person who knows he needs dental care and wants to have attractive, healthy teeth. In other words, he is motivated to approach a dentist. At the same time, he is fearful of going to the dentist and wants to avoid the experience. These two competing tendencies, one to approach and one to avoid, leave the person in a state of conflict. Dollard and Miller further found through their research that the two tendencies change in strength as the person in conflict moves closer to or farther from the desired but feared situation. As one is farther away in time or distance, the approach tendency is stronger than the avoidance tendency. But as one nears the feared situation, the avoidance tendency increases in strength more quickly than does the approach tendency. This situation is illustrated in Figure 1-1. The lines called *goal gradients* in this figure represent the different approach and avoidance tendencies. The slope of the gradient going from "close" to "far" from the goal is different for the two tenden- cies. When the person is far away from the goal, the approach tendency is higher or stronger than the avoidance. As he moves closer, he reaches a point where the two tendencies are of equal strength (where the gradients intersect). At this point, the person is torn by two equally strong tendencies. If the person were placed closer to the dentist's office, the avoidance tendency would be stronger, causing him to retreat. But as he got past the intersection, the approach tendency would be strongest. He is caught between these competing response tendencies. This conceptualization can help explain a common occurrence among fearful patients and one that causes dentists and their staffs many problems: patients cancel- ling or not appearing for appointments they have made. When the appointment is far off, say three weeks away, the approach tendency is stronger than the avoidance and the person is able to call for an appointment. It doesn't seem so bad at a distance. He may have

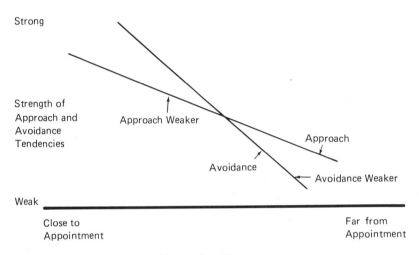

FIGURE 1-1. Approach-Avoidance Conflict

some anxiety, but his desire for needed dental care is stronger. As the time draws closer to the actual appointment, the avoidance tendency becomes stronger than the approach tendency. At this point, the anxiety becomes too strong to resist and the person does not "show." The result is that the dentist is frustrated because he has a vacancy in his schedule. The patient too may feel frustrated with himself for "being such a coward" and for not getting the dental care he needs and wants.

In order to break this cycle of approaching and avoiding, something must intervene to lower the avoidance gradient or to raise the approach gradient. For example, if a fearful person who has avoided or cancelled several prophylactic appointments because of fear develops a severe toothache, the pain may be enough to raise the approach gradient sufficiently to exceed the avoidance tendency. Or a fearful patient may meet a dentist socially and find her to be a concerned and caring person, very different from the patient's previous image of dentists. The changed attitude about dentists' concern for patients may be sufficient to lower the avoidance gradient. Later chapters of this book are devoted to these goals:

decreasing the fear and avoidance gradient and increasing the motivation or approach gradient. For now, let's turn to a classification system that describes some of the types of fearful patients seen in dental practice, using the approach-avoidance concepts.

The types of patients we describe serve mainly for illustrative purposes; and their typology should not be taken as a diagnostic system. However, practitioners who have worked with fearful or apprehensive patients will be able to classify many of them by using these categories.

Apprehensive Patients

This classification encompasses the largest group of patients who experience some degree of dental fear. The term "apprehensive" is used to describe them because the fear they experience is relatively

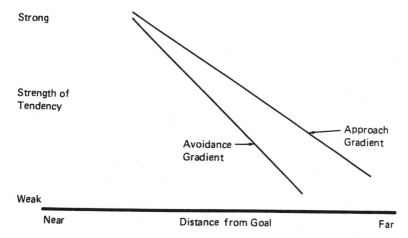

FIGURE 1-2. *Approach-Avoidance Gradient for the Apprehensive Patient*

moderate and does not lead toavoidance or necessarily cause significant treatment problems. The situation is graphically displayed in Figure 1-2. Using the approach-avoidance concepts, we see that the approach gradient is higher than the avoidance gradient, allowing the person to appear at the office. However, by the time the patient arrives, the avoidance gradient comes very close to intersecting and the patient begins to experience some fear.

Apprehensive patients will experience some discomfort both in anticipation of an appointment and while in the dental office. They may say to themselves, "I hope he doesn't find any cavities," or "I hope this is quick," or "Hope this won't hurt." Similar statements may be made to the dentist or assistant, but often with a nervous type of humor. This patient presents hardly any problem to the provider. He is generally cooperative and may successfully mask apprehension for fear of looking "childish." In fact, many patients within this category have successfully masked their fear to the extent that the dentist may have no idea that they are experiencing any emotional upset. It is important to note, however, that many such apprehensive patients may be potential phobic patients. If they experience sufficient pain or discomfort or believe that they have not been treated well, their fear may increase enough to raise their avoidance gradient. The result might be that they seek a new dentist who will be more attentive to their general comfort or avoid dentistry altogether. In later sections of this book we will discuss procedures dental personnel can use to identify such patients."Goers but Haters"

Patients in this category also make appointments on a relatively regular basis but experience considerably more intense fear than does the apprehensive patient. They may begin their worrying days in advance of their appointment. As the appointment day approaches, their approach and avoidance gradients come closer and closer to intersecting, as the fear rises (see Figure 1-3). However, once the appointment is set, they feel a strong obligation to follow through with it. This motivation keeps their approach gradient enough above their avoidance gradient to ensure that they appear at the office.

As can be seen in Figure 1-3, the approach avoidance gradients are not too different from those of the Apprehensive Patient. The main factor differentiating them is that the avoidance gradient is steeper. However, the approach gradient is also high because of a commitment to appear once an appointment has been made.

Once patients are in the office, their fear level causes them considerable discomfort, and they are less able to hide or mask it. They may tell the dentist directly that they "hate dentistry," and cause problems for the dentist. Such patients often stop the dentist, frequently need to be told to "open wider," "to relax," etc. This in turn causes considerable stress for the dentist, who knows that the patient is reacting to him or his treatment. Such patients require

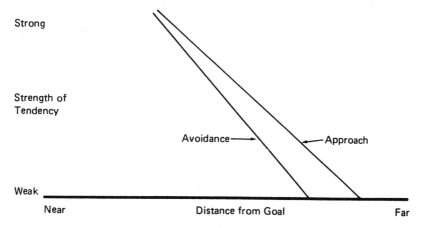

FIGURE 1-3. *Approach-Avoidance Gradient for the "Goer but Hater"*

more time to treat and often cause the dentist to get behind schedule, further increasing his stress. The result is an unpleasant experience for both patient and dentist.

Partial Avoiders

Patients classified as partial avoiders are similar in many respects to the "goers but haters." However, their fear causes them to put off making appointments for years at a time. If their fear is not treated, they are unlikely to become regular dental patients. In other words, their avoidance tendency is considerably stronger than their approach tendency, and they continue to avoid dentistry as long as possible (see Figure 1-4).

At some point, other factors intervene to raise the approach gradient (as depicted by the dotted line in Figure 1-4). Typical factors motivating them to approach are urging by family members who may actually make the appointment or the occurrence of some dental problem that renders their discomfort greater than their fear.

The emotional suffering they experience is similar in intensity to that of the "goer but hater," but the anticipatory discomfort lasts longer. Because of the length of time between appointments, partial avoiders may require rather extensive treatment. They require longer times to treat because of both the fear and neglect, further

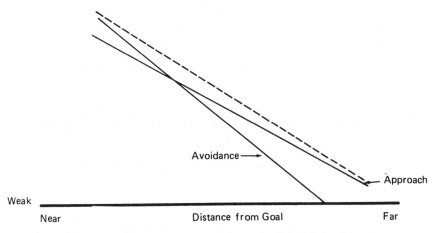

FIGURE 1-4. *Approach-Avoidance Gradient for Partial Avoiders*

increasing their discomfort. Stress experienced by the dentist is similar to that noted for dentists treating the "goer but hater."

Total Avoiders

Total avoiders are rarely seen in dental offices. They avoid dentistry at all costs. Their main contact with dentistry is through emergency clinics where they may appear in excruciating pain. Their avoidance gradient is well above their approach gradient and the two rarely intersect (see Figure 1-5).

Such patients will often tolerate very high levels of dental pain rather than submit to even emergency dental care, even though the pain from the dental problem far exceeds what they might experience at the hands of the dentist. This extreme avoidance, clearly irrational and interfering with daily functioning, qualifies as a phobia.

Persons with extreme dental phobias often self-medicate. They use alcohol or other pain-killing drugs and not uncommonly will be under the influence of these substances when they appear at an emergency clinic. Many see the ultimate solution to their problems as having all their teeth extracted under general anesthesia. It is exceedingly difficult to treat patients presenting such intense fear and pain. Unless treated for their fear, they are unlikely to return for subsequent appointments.

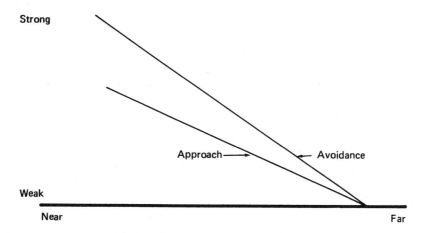

FIGURE 1-5. *Approach-Avoidance Gradient forTotal Avoiders*

What are the clinical implications of approach avoidance gradients? Dentists typically try to increase the "approach" by extolling the benefits of treatment. The problem with this strategy is that fearful patients are generally very aware of the benefits of treatment. The problem is that they do not believe they can tolerate it. Consequently, the strategies that we will discuss throughout this book will focus primarily on lowering the avoidance barriers.

PREVALENCE OF DENTAL FEAR

Throughout our lives, few of us are immune from some form of fear or anxiety problem. However, one of the most prevalent fears is of dentistry. Through numerous recent studies of the prevalence of dental fears we have acquired a firm understanding of its extent throughout most of the world.

One of the earliest studies sampled the prevalence of various fears in the residents of a moderate size New England community and found that fear of dentists was the fifth most common fear reported (Agras *et al.*, 1969). The investigators found that 19.8 percent of the population reported some moderate degree of fear. In further categorizing fears of a more severe nature, they found that an additional 2.4 percent reported "intense" fear of dentistry, implying that some degree of dental avoidance due to fear was present in this population.

In another large-scale study surveying a random sample of the U.S. population, approximately 6 percent of the respondents reported not receiving needed dental care because of fear (Friedson & Feldman, 1958).

Kleinknecht and associates (1984) obtained questionnaire data from some 920 persons concerning their fear and avoidance of dentistry. Although not a random sample, the respondents were from two geographically distinct populations (the states of Florida and Washington) and were of a broad age distribution ranging from 14 to 83 years of age. The questionnaire, called the *Dental Fear Survey*, will be described in detail in Chapter 4. For now, let us look at the responses to three of the questions that pertain to fear and patterns of avoidance. The first question asked was: "Has fear of dentistry ever caused you to put off making an appointment?" Table 1-1 shows the percentages of respondents who indicated each of the five response alternatives. As can be seen in the right-hand column headed "Total," 44.5 percent of the respondents indicated that they had put off making an appointment at least once because of fear, and 4.7 percent reported doing so "nearly every time" they felt they should make an appointment.

TABLE 1-1
Percentages of Respondents Who Report Having Put Off
Making a Dental Appointment Because of Fear

Response	Male	Female.	Total
	%	%	%
"Never"	60.8	50.0	55.5
"Once or Twice"	19.3	20.6	19.9
"A Few Times"	9.3	12.1	10.7
"Often"	7.7	9.9	9.0
"Nearly Every Time"	2.8	6.3	4.7

n = 920

The second question, which addresses a somewhat more severe situation, asked: "Has fear ever caused you to cancel or not appear for an appointment that was already made?" Table 1-2 shows that, overall, 14.1 percent reported doing this at least once, and nearly 2 percent reported cancelling either "often" or "nearly every time." These figures, however, may be an underestimate of the actual prevalence of avoidance because the majority of respondents were active patients of dentists who cooperated in this study. A study from Sweden reports that 14 percent of a sample felt dental visits to be "so uncomfortable that they were unable to follow through with treatment" (Seeman & Molin, 1975).

TABLE 1-2
Percentages of Respondents Who Report Having Canceled or
Not Appeared for a Dental Appointment Because of Fear

Response	Male	Female	Total
	%	%	%
"Never"	90.0	82.3	85.9
"Once or Twice"	7.2	9.5	8.4
"A Few Times"	2.3	4.6	3.6
"Often"	0.5	2.4	1.5
"Nearly Every Time"	0.0	0.8	0.4

n = 920

Another question from this survey asked: "All things considered, how fearful are you of having dental work done?" The results of this question, shown in Table 1-3, indicate as stated previously that 74.6

percent reported having at least "a little" fear of dentistry. Further, we can see that 17.5 percent reported their fear to be "much" or "very much." This figure compares closely to that reported by Agras and associates (1969).

TABLE 1-3
Percentage of Respondents Answering the Question:
"All Things Considered, How Fearful Are You of Having Dental Work Done?"

Response	Male	Female	Total
	%	%	%
"Not at all"	29.1	21.8	25.4
"A little"	40.3	32.7	36.6
"Somewhat"	19.6	21.6	20.5
"Much"	6.1	13.7	10.2
"Very much"	4.0	10.1	7.3

n = 920

A more recent population based study (Milgrom *et al.*, 1988) assessed dental fear in 1,019 randomly selected adults in Seattle, Washington. Of all respondents, 50 percent reported some fear of the dentist, with 28 percent acknowledging being a little afraid, 13.1 percent being somewhat afraid, 4.3 percent being very afraid, and 3.0 percent being terrified of dental treatment. The prevalence figure for clinically significant fears in Seattle during 1986 was 204 adults per 1,000 population.

Similar findings have been published regarding Dutch adults over 16 years of age (Stouthard & Hoogstraten, 1990); Singapore children, adolescents, and university students (Chellappah *et al.*, 1990; Teo *et al.*, 1990; Milgrom *et al.*, 1990; Milgrom *et al.*, 1992); and Japanese students (Domoto *et al.*, 1988).

A somewhat lower, but nevertheless significant, prevalence of fears was reported in urban Sweden (Hakeberg *et al.*, 1992); in Dallas, Texas (Gatchel, 1989); in Finnish children (Alvesalo *et al.*, 1993); and among university students in Brazil (Cesar *et al.*, 1993). A review of many of these and similar studies and a discussion of some of the methodological problems in comparing them has been published by ter Horst & de Wit (1993).

These data clearly indicate that dental fear is a widespread occurrence with consequences for patient health and dental practice. The Seattle data show a relationship between high dental fear and the length of time since the last dental visit. Approximately 59 percent of the high-fear groups had seen a dentist within the last 12 months, compared with more than 77 percent of the low-fear individuals. More importantly, among the high-fear group, more than 24 percent had not seen a dentist in more than two years. Moreover, over half of the high-fear sample reported delays in making appointments and nearly one in ten people failed to appear for scheduled appointments "often" or "nearly every time."

Similar results are found for school children (Milgrom *et al.*, 1994). Thus, a sizeable segment of the general population that could benefit from dental care does not receive that care because of fear.

PREVALENCE RATES BY AGE AND SEX

In the previous section, the various rates and percentages of persons expressing dental fear reflect the general population. However, within the general population there are some differences in dental fear related to age and gender.

Age Differences in Fear Prevalence

As we look at older populations, we find a lower prevalence of fear associated with dentistry, as is true of most other forms of fears and phobias.

The available data show that most fears begin in the pre-teen years (Agras *et al.*, 1969; Kleinknecht *et al.*, 1973; Bernstein & Klein-knecht, 1979; Milgrom *et al.*, 1988). Fortunately, many of these fears lessen with a person's increasing experience and maturity (Locker *et al.*, 1991). Unfortunately, some people's dental fear persists into adulthood, and people can also develop fear of the dentist during adulthood.

To provide an overview on the relation between age and the presence and intensity of dental fear, we can look at the figures shown in Table 1-4. This table shows the percentages of 317 persons, grouped into five different age levels, who indicated their degree of dental fear. The scale used here is the one used in Table 1-3.

The left-hand column of Table 1-4 shows a clear trend: as we go from younger age groups to the older, there is an increasing percentage of respondents who indicate that they have no fear of dentistry. In the 14-to-21-year-old group, 7.7 percent indicate no fear, while that figure rises to 53.7 percent in the group from 50 to 83 years of age.

Looking at the far right-hand column, which indicates the percentage who report "very much" fear, we see this trend reversed. Here, 23.1 percent of the youngest age group report "very much" fear while only 3.0 percent of the oldest group indicate this much fear.

If we were to rely only on the overall figures concerning the percentages of persons who report being fearful, we would get a distorted picture. For instance

TABLE 1-4
Percentages of Respondents
From Five Age Levels Who Indicated Their Degree of Dental Fear

	Fear Level					
Age Level	*None At All* %	*A Little* %	*Some* %	*Much* %	*Very Much* %	*Total* %
14-21	7.7	50.0	11.5	7.7	23.1	100
n = 26						
22-29	23.1	32.7	18.3	17.3	3.7	100
n = 104						
30-39	34.6	29.6	13.6	11.1	11.1	100
n=81						
40-49	35.9	46.2	10.3	5.1	2.6	100
n = 39						
50-83	53.7	29.0	10.4	3.0	3.0	100
n = 67						
Total %	32.8	34.4	13.9	10.4	8.5	100

n = 317

from the sample of patients shown in Table 1-4, the bottom row shows, overall, only 8.5 percent indicating the highest level of fear. This is considerably lower than is true for the youngest group, and much too high for older groups.

In addition to the questionnaire survey data just presented, there are other indictions that older patients, in general, experience less fear than do their younger counterparts. This information comes from a study in which patients were evaluated for signs of fear while they were in a dental office and undergoing treatment (Klein-knecht & Bernstein, 1978). It was found that patients over 40 years of age, compared with those 40 and under, experienced less anxiety during an appointment, reported that before treatment they ex-pected to experience less pain, and actually experienced less pain (during treatment) and less physiological arousal as indicated by measures of their sweating response.

Although the data demonstrate that older patients experience less fear than do younger patients, keep in mind that these are only general trends and there are many exceptions. We cannot assume that simply because a patient is older, he or she will not be fearful, or that all younger patients will be fearful.

Gender Differences in Fear Prevalence

In dental fear, as with most specific fears and phobias, females generally report being somewhat more fearful than do males. These findings have been borne out in survey questionnaire studies of samples taken from the general population (Agras *et al.*, 1969; Milgrom *et al.*, 1988; Stouthard & Hoogstraten, 1990; Neverlien, 1990; Hakeberg *et al.*, 1992); young people and college students in the U.S. and abroad (Kleinknecht *et al.*, 1973; Corah *et al.*, 1978; Bernstein & Kleinknecht, 1979; Bernstein & Kleinknecht, 1982; Nippert & Meier, 1987; Frazer & Hampson, 1988; Brauner, 1989; Teo *et al.*, 1990; Schwarz, 1990; De Jongh *et al.*, 1991; Mellor, 1992; Milgrom *et al.*, 1994), and dental patients (Kleinknecht & Bernstein, 1978; Vervoorn *et al.*, 1989).

The prevalence data previously reported in Tables 1-1, 1-2, and 1-3 show the percentage of males versus females who report varying degrees of dental fear. As can be seen, males predominate in responding to the "not at all" or "never" categories for having put off making an appointment, not appearing for an appointment once made, and general dental fear. Conversely, females are more frequently represented in the response categories indicating greater fear and avoidance.

Similar findings are reported showing females to exhibit more palmar sweating than males when viewing a film of a dental operation (Bernstein & Kleinknecht, 1982), and while undergoing dental treatment (Weisenberg *et al.*, 1976; Kleinknecht & Bernstein, 1978; Smith *et al.*, 1987; Roy-Byrne *et al.*, 1994).

Although the data reported here consistently find females to demonstrate more dental fear than do males, the differences are typically not of such magnitude that one could reliably make individual predictions about which patients are going to be fearful based only on their gender. Nonetheless, there is an overwhelming preponderance of females among patients seeking treatment for dental fear. The percentages of females in such programs range from 75 percent to 86 percent (Shaw & Thoresen, 1974; Bernstein & Kleinknecht, 1978; Klepac *et al.*, 1982). These figures are consistent with our experience at the University of Washington Dental Fears Clinic. The fact that females are more likely than males to seek treatment for their fear should not be too surprising. Women also are the more frequent users of dental services in general.

OBJECTS AND SITUATIONS FEARED

In the preceding section, we discussed dental fear as though the whole concept of dentistry is feared. Although this is the case for some, most people are able to identify specific aspects of dentistry that frighten them most and least. In this section, we describe those situations and procedures that patients report as being most fear arousing. These elements are classified into two general categories: (1) specific situations, instruments, and procedures which are feared, and (2) characteristics of dental personnel that patients find disturbing.

Situations, Instruments, and Procedures

Two instruments are consistently cited by patients as producing the most fear or dread: the anesthetic syringe, or "needle," and the "drill." Among virtually all studies conducted that ask patients to rank or rate the elements of dentistry most feared, these two instruments come out first and second (Gale, 1972; Kleinknecht *et al.*, 1973; Bernstein *et al.*, 1979; Milgrom *et al.*, 1988). The results of one representative study are shown in Table 1-5. Two hundred students were asked to indicate the amount of fear they experienced when confronted with each of the twelve situations listed. The table shows the average rating (on a 5-point scale) of the amount of fear produced by each of these situations, along with the ranking from most (1) to least (5) fearful. Overall, the *feel* of the syringe was rated number 1; very close behind was the *sight* of the needle.

The next most fear-provoking aspect of dentistry, ranked number 3, was the sound of the drill, followed by the feeling or vibration from it. The relative ranking of these stimuli holds true whether the respondent reports being highly fearful or not. Although the intensity of fear is greater for the high-fear person, the relative ranking remains the same. This has similarly been found for males and females where females rate each item as causing more fear, but each item holds the same relative position compared to the other items.

TABLE 1-5
Patient Ratings of Fear-Provoking Qualities of
Dental Instruments and Procedures

	Total		High Fear		Low Fear	
	Mean	*Rank*	*Mean*	*Rank*	*Mean*	*Rank*
Feel the "needle"	3.40	1	4.14	1	2.01	1
See the "needle"	3.31	2	4.08	2.5	2.80	2
Hear the "drill"	3.25	3	4.08	2.5	2.70	3

	Total		High Fear		Low Fear	
	Mean	*Rank*	*Mean*	*Rank*	*Mean*	*Rank*
Feel the "drill"	3.21	4	4.05	4	2.00	4
See the "drill"	2.92	5	3.88	5	2.32	5
Being seated in operatory	2.57	0	3.51	7	1.95	7
Waiting room	2.48	7	3.36	0	1.89	8
Office smell	2.43	8	3.10	6	1.96	6
Seeing dentist	2.39	0	3.30	8	2.78	9
Approaching office	2.20	10	3.10	10	1.00	11
Prophylaxis	1.89	11	2.30	12	1.02	10
Making appointment	1.75	12	2.34	11	1.35	12

Rating scale: 1 = no fear, 2 = a little, 3 = some, 4 = much, 5 = very much

It has also been shown that the injection produces the most physical fear reaction, such as increased heart rate (Hewitt & Stricker, 1977) and increased palmar sweating response (Kleinknecht & Bernstein, 1978; Bernstein & Kleinknecht, 1982).

The fear-provoking qualities of the other elements associated with a dental appointment are also of interest. For the most part, the rankings increase the closer one gets to the actual treatment itself. This is an example of the approach-avoidance gradients described earlier. Far from the feared situation, such as when one makes an appointment, the avoidance is less intense than the approach

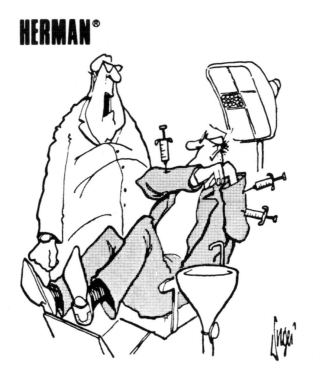

HERMAN®

"WILL YOU KEEP YOUR ARMS DOWN!"

tendency. When approaching the office, smelling the office, sitting in the waiting room, and being seated in the operatory, the fear and avoidance increase. If the person's fear becomes too great, his avoidance gradient becomes steeper. The person may not keep the appointment, which didn't seem so fearful when he merely arranged it.

The relative rankings of the fear-producing qualities of this sequence of events and specific stimuli hold true whether the person doing the rating is highly fearful or not (Gale, 1972; Kleinknecht *et al.*, 1973; Bernstein & Kleinknecht, 1979). Only the rated intensity of the fear changes. Similarly, males and females tend to rank the situations in the same order, although, as noted earlier, females tend to rate these situations as somewhat more fearful than males.

It should be noted that while these rankings are generally true for most people, there are many important individual exceptions. For example, we have encountered some patients whose fear is primarily of the sensations associated with drilling. But these same patients see the anesthetic syringe as highly positive because they know the anesthesia will decrease the aversive effects of the drilling. We have seen others who experience virtually no fear of any part of dentistry except that when the anesthetic is about to be injected they become very fearful and defensive. They are quite specifically needle phobic. School children are often fearful of choking and of having strangers touch them in addition to their fears of injections and drilling (Milgrom *et al.*, 1994).

Although these rankings are important for understanding dental fear in general, one cannot assume that each patient has the same problem. Each patient must be evaluated individually for his own unique pattern of fears (Liddell *et al.*, 1994). Chapter 4 will discuss such individual assessment.

Dental Personnel

The Dentist. To patients, whether fearful or not, the dentist is clearly the most salient feature in the dental office. As noted previously, the "needle" and "drill" are the most feared specific stimuli. However, some patients may view these as extensions of the dentist and they influence the patients' perception of the dentist. For others, it is the dentist's professional behavior and personal characteristics which are critically important in influencing a patient's views of dentistry.

Information about the impact of the dentist on patients comes from a study in which a large number of college students were asked to describe all the factors that contributed to their attitude toward dentistry (Kleinknecht *et al.*, 1979). Most common were those that directly referred to the personal and professional behavior of the dentist. Indeed, 91 percent of all respondents made some direct comments about the dentist affecting their attitudes. This focus was present whether the respondent was male or female and whether he or she reported being fearful or not.

The results showed that among those who considered themselves fearful, 50 percent had negative things to say about the dentist. Among the low-fear group, 30 percent had negative comments. The general focus of these negative comments reflected two themes. One centered on personal attributes of the dentist, such as "he is impersonal," "nasty," "disinterested," "nervous," "mean," "uncaring," and "cold." The second theme related to what was called "professional behavior" and included comments such as "he is incompetent," "rough," "he yells at me," "would not stop drilling when I told him it hurt," "told me it wouldn't hurt when it really would," "he would strap my arms and legs down." Such comments were succinctly characterized by one of our fearful patients who described his dentist as having the "demeanor of a linebacker and touch of a jackhammer."

It is also of interest to compare patients' reports of pain during treatment relative to comments about the dentist. Although pain is often considered the reason that people avoid dentistry, the situation may not be so clear cut. In the study noted above, half of the fearful patients cited the dentist as an important factor in their negative attitudes. Of these, 81 percent did *not* cite pain as affecting their attitudes. For these patients, the dentist himself had greater impact on their fear than did pain.

Further supporting the personal impact of the dentist were the comments made by many of the fearless patients that were in stark contrast to the negative statements cited above. Non-fearful patients, even those who reported having experienced some pain, indicated a strong personal liking for their dentist with comments such as: "He is patient, careful, friendly, polite, skilled, professional, warm, and caring." We will have more to say concerning these comments about the dentist in Chapter 2 when we discuss the development of dental fear and avoidance.

The Dental Auxiliary. In contrast to the dentist, the auxiliary personnel were mentioned considerably less often as influencing patients' attitudes toward dentistry. Among the 28 percent who did mention auxiliaries, most commented positively. It is interesting that the majority of the positive comments were made by males who reported themselves as being fearful, whereas the few negative comments were made by female patients. Apparently, auxiliary personnel are seen by most patients as a positive, soothing, and non-threatening aspect of dentistry. Auxiliaries help create the atmosphere in an office. Their early contact with the patient may be very important in creating patient comfort. As in the treatment of children (Weinstein *et al.*, 1983), the assistant is often underutilized in fear treatment. In the Dental Fears Research Clinic at the University of Washington and in private practice (Kroeger, 1987), a well-trained dental hygienist or dental assistant often provides much of the fear-reduction needed for people with specific phobias.

Fear of Being Embarrassed and Belittled

Less common, but significant, is the fear some patients express about being embarrassed and belittled by dental personnel. The importance of this fear as a cause of dental avoidance was shown in a study by Gale (1972), who found that among 25 situations rated for their fear-producing qualities, the statement, "Dentist tells you that you have bad teeth," was ranked third. In this study, anticipation of such comments was found to be more fear provoking than receiving an injection. Also in this list of 25 situations was the statement: "Dentist laughs as he looks in your mouth," which was ranked as the seventh most fear producing. Although the percentage of cases in which these concerns are found varies from one study to the next, most find that a significant proportion of patients report fear of personal criticism by the dentist (Foresberg, 1966; Kleinknecht *et al.*, 1973). Such comments by dentists are neither personally nor professionally appropriate and can affect not only the patients' fear and avoidance of dentistry but more generally the public's attitude toward the entire profession.

Patient Vulnerability and Loss of Control

A final factor related to patient fear and avoidance is the sense of
personal vulnerability and lack of control over the dentist. It is a
basic tenet of psychology that people under stress experience fear in
a potentially threatening situation in which they have little or no
control (Seligman, 1975; Miller, 1979; Davis & Neale, 1981). In a
stressful situation, the extent to which they have or, *think* they have,
some personal control over the stressor, there is a corresponding
lessening of fear. If pain is involved, the amount of control affects
the extent to which pain will be judged as more or less aversive.

We believe that this situation has great relevance to patients' reaction to dentistry. Consider, from the patient's point of view, what
typically transpires during dental treatment. First, the patient is
brought into an operatory, which contains many shining, sharp, and
unfamiliar instruments that she vaguely knows might hurt her. She
is then reclined in a chair with her head lower than her feet, a very
unaccustomed and awkward position, and one that makes it difficult
to move the whole body, or to escape. Then, a rubber dam is
placed—which prevents her from being able to use speech, the
accustomed means of avoiding harm. Further (and possibly more
fear provoking), is that with the rubber dam, many patients may
have difficulty breathing until they learn they must breathe through
the nose. This may be particularly frightening for those who have
had no previous experience with a rubber dam and those who have
respiratory problems such as asthma. Finally, imagine looking up to
see the dentist and assistant hovering, holding instruments. In this
highly unnatural and restrictive situation, it is not surprising that a
person feels vulnerable. The patient is virtually at the mercy of the
dentist who is in the position of control and power. Particularly for
apprehensive patients, the perception of the dentist as a powerful
professional who is in charge inhibits them from making requests
that might increase their comfort. They may feel that it is not their
place to question authority.

Given this vulnerability, consider how imposing the instruments
and the dentist must appear. It is little wonder that some 75 percent
of patients feel at least some fear under these conditions.

Because the dentist must ultimately maintain some control over
the situation in order to carry out the treatment, he cannot turn over

full control to the patient. In fact, it is not necessary to put the patient in control in order to reduce her fear. Numerous studies have shown that the critical element is that the patient *believes* he has some control over the potential threat. Therefore, if the dentist can convince the patient through words and actions that he can terminate the procedure if it becomes too aversive, less fear and less pain are likely to be experienced. And the patient's need for exercising any control will also be lessened. Enhancing patients' feeling of control is one of several techniques to be discussed in greater detail in later chapters dealing with treatment and prevention of dental fear.

CONCLUSION

In this first chapter, we have attempted to describe the problem of dental fear, its extent in the general population, and some of the factors from which this fear derives. We noted that up to 75 percent of the population may experience some fear, but that about 10 percent are adversely affected to the extent that they avoid dentistry, to the detriment of their oral health.

The sight and sensations of the syringe and the drill were shown to be the specific elements most cited as fear provoking. However, the greatest overall impact on patients centers around the perception of control and the personal and professional characteristics of the dentist.

It is also important to remember that there are rational and irrational elements in most cases of dental fear. The fear reaction is rational to the extent that some pain and discomfort may result. However, we often see reactions that far exceed what would normally be expected under the circumstances of typical dental treatment. When you consider these seemingly irrational reactions, it is important to view them in their historical contexts. What have the patients' past experiences been with dentistry? How do they currently perceive the dental situation? Even though a patient's fear may seem irrational at the present (such as having a panic attack while he is undergoing a simple prophylaxis), the fear may be viewed in a different light when we learn of the patient's early experiences.

The current treatment situation may pose little real threat to the patient, but ultimately what determines the reaction will be the patient's *perception* or *belief* concerning what might occur. To the extent that the dentist can understand patients' perceptions and where they come from, their seemingly irrational behavior will be more understandable. Then the dentist will be in a position to begin changing patients' negative perceptions and expectations in ways that are more adaptive and health promoting.

In the process of working to change fearful patients' expectations, it is important that the dentist realize that most fearful patients are, in most other aspects of their lives, rational, normal, and productive individuals. The presence by itself of a seemingly irrational reaction to dentistry should not be taken to imply that the patient is more generally fearful, neurotic, or personally weak.

We believe that it is most productive and accurate to view the fearful dental patient and the problems posed by the fear in the same way the dentist views dental disease. That is, the problem is identified and diagnosed, and a rational treatment plan is followed to remedy the problem. All of these therapeutic processes are based on current scientific knowledge. In the chapters that follow, these processes are presented.

QUESTIONS AND EXERCISES

1. Construct and describe an approach-avoidance gradient for a fear-inducing or anxiety-provoking situation in *your own life.*

2. About what percentage of the general population reports being very afraid or terrified of dental treatment. What percentage reports being only "a little" or not fearful of treatment?

3. What interpersonal aspects of dental professionals do patients report as significantly influencing their feelings about treatment?

4. What two aspects of dental treatment do patients report as causing them the most anxiety in dentistry. For each item listed, describe what you as a dental professional could do to reduce their fear or apprehension.

TWO

Etiology of Dental Fear

- Direct and Indirect Experiences
- Helplessness and Control
- A Model of Fear Acquisition
- A Model of Fear Treatment

People are not born fearful. The association of fear with dentistry develops out of socialization and personal learning experiences. Some of these experiences come from direct contact with dentistry while others are communicated indirectly through other people and the mass media.

As noted in Chapter 1, the capacity to experience fear is an inborn characteristic. Our nervous systems are "wired" in such a way that we perceive and interpret threatening events and react physiologically and behaviorally to escape and avoid dangers. However, the development of fear to dental stimuli occurs through learning processes. First, we will describe each of the processes separately, and then we will present a general model integrating these processes as they typically combine in many cases of dental fear. Finally, we will discuss the implications that this fear development model has for prevention and treatment or "unlearning" of dental fear.

Current thinking argues that although fears are often acquired as a function of direct experience, they may also be acquired through two other pathways, vicarious experiences related to or observed as threatening information (Rachman, 1990). Ollendick and King (1991) examined ten common fears in a large multinational sample of children and adolescents and found that most of the people attributed the onset of their fears to vicarious and instructional factors, often combined with direct experience. Öst (1987) has suggested that as many as 80 percent of clinically significant fears are acquired directly. In recent work with low-income mothers and children in Seattle, we found that both direct experience and the mothers' fears and poor experiences communicated to the children were strong, independent predictors of fear. This was true even after we controlled for gender, age, race, and other factors that might also affect the relationship to fear development (Milgrom *et al.*, 1994).

DIRECT EXPERIENCES LEADING TO DENTAL FEAR

The most common way patients develop fear and avoidance of dentistry is through direct negative experience in the dental office. These negative experiences may take the form of intense pain or fright, or they may involve negative interpersonal interactions between dentist and patient. In either case, the patient forms an association between some aspect of dentistry and unpleasant experiences. These profound associations can develop from a single dental experience.

Conditioned Emotional Responses

We present the following case description of one of our fearful patient's reported experiences with dentistry to illustrate how direct experiences can lead to fear and avoidance.

> Nora recalled that her early dental experiences were painful and she did not like going at all. However, her parents continued to take her to the dentist on a relatively regular basis. Later, as a 26-year-old adult, Nora experienced an incident that firmly set her into the category of Avoider.
>
> "One day the dentist was filling one of my teeth and accidentally broke off part of another tooth. This really upset me but I knew that I had to go back to get it fixed. At this appointment, the drill slipped from my tooth and drilled a hole in my tongue. I never went back."

Intensely painful and frightening experiences such as this often result in what is called *Conditioned Emotional Responses* (CER). Figure 2-1 shows diagrammatically how a Conditioned Emotional Response can develop. A CER is a conditioned response that has a strong emotional component. It develops when an intensely negative or painful stimulus causes a reflexive emotional response. The negative experience, however, does not occur in isolation. It occurs typically in the presence of some other stimuli with which it becomes associated. The initial stimulus causing pain is called an *Unconditioned Stimulus* (US) because it automatically causes a response, pain or fear. This automatic response is referred to as an *Unconditioned Response* (UR). The UR can elicit an emotional response itself, even without the original painful or frightening stimulation (US). This latter, associated stimulus is called a *Conditioned Stimulus* (CS). The CS then, by itself, acquires the capacity to elicit an emotional response causing the person to experience arousal and avoidance behavior.

In the case described above, the dentist, or dentistry in general, became a CS for Nora which caused her to be upset at even the thought of "dentist," and she actively avoided contact with dentistry. We could say that this experience caused her dental avoidance gradient to become higher than her approach gradient.

The CER, which a person develops by associating pain with another stimulus, causes her to avoid such encounters again. The strength of the CER will depend on her evaluation of the US (Davey, 1989). This is important because a series of successful visits, as when children are exposed to dentistry slowly, can inoculate a patient against developing fear when a particularly painful visit is unavoidable. When fearful reactions are severe, they are beyond the individual's immediate control. Even though rationally Nora might know that the prospects of being hurt as she was at her last visit are relatively remote, the emotional reaction is still there, automatically. No one, including herself, could talk her out of experiencing the CER.

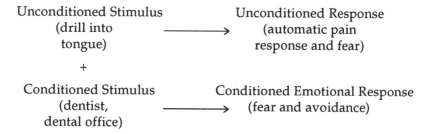

FIGURE 2-1. A Conditioned Emotional Response to Dentistry

An additional factor enters at this point, which can actually make the CER stronger, even without re-exposure to the US. As noted above, the person may have a fearful response at the thought of going to the dentist. That is, the CS, the thought of a dentist, elicits the emotional response.

When one avoids or escapes from an unpleasant situation, the result is reinforcing: that is, one feels relief. This reinforcement then further serves to keep the person away from the CS. By not thinking about dentistry, he avoids the CS and feels less anxiety. Unfortunately, this keeps him from returning to the dentist where he can actually find out that all experiences are not like the one which caused the CER to begin with. As we will discuss later, one of the best ways to eliminate the CER is to gradually re-expose the person to the CS (dental situation) without his experiencing the UR (pain).

Repeated non-traumatic exposures tend to eliminate the CER.

Dentist Behavior and Patients' Perceptions

In the preceding section, we showed how the conditioning process can elicit reflexive reactions in the patient, based on the association of painful or frightening stimuli with a person or object that is also present. Such associations are relatively automatic and require no intent. However, as shown in Chapter 1, not all fearful patients report significant painful experiences of this sort, yet they fear and avoid dentistry. Recall that a large percentage felt that the personal and professional characteristics of the *dentist* were responsible for their fear, independent of pain.

The direct experiences here are of an interpersonal nature. Some fearful patients described their dentists as harsh, uncaring, insulting, or belittling. Interpersonal characteristics are the primary basis on which we form friendships. We prefer to associate with people who are interested in us and who try to make us feel comfortable and at ease. We avoid people who make fun of us, insult us, yell at us, and who hurt us physically or psychologically.

One of our patients described how the behavior of several of his early dentists contributed to his later avoidance. Marvin was self-conscious about his teeth because, as he described them, they were "... ugly, irregular and not white."

> I remember one dentist as having bad breath. I only went when it was absolutely necessary. Making an appointment would take me weeks and going would produce a strange dizziness. Being there was worse because the dentist would look at my teeth rather disgustingly and would make nasty remarks. Any pain I ever felt was really of less importance than my fear of being embarrassed and humiliated.

For Marvin, the avoidance and his fear reaction were determined on the basis of his dentist's interpersonal behavior toward him. He felt the pain was of less consequence.

The simple rules of interpersonal liking and disliking apply strongly with dentistry. From the patients' point of view, much more is at stake than just being in the presence of the dentist. As patients, we are captive to the dentist, and many of us feel that we have little choice in what happens to us once we are in the chair and the rubber dam is placed. Under these conditions, we need to trust the person wielding the potentially harmful instruments. And if that person has not treated us in a manner conducive to liking and trust, we may generalize our concerns to question how he or she will treat us physically. "If he treated me badly with his words and manner, how will he treat my body?" "If she is not concerned with me personally, will she be concerned with how I feel physically?" "If he is clumsy personally, will he be clumsy with his hands?" *Trust* is a major issue for many who fear and avoid dental treatment.

HERMAN®

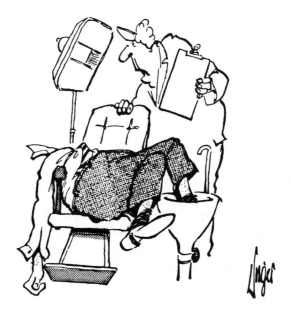

"Dr. Burns says you need two more appointments."

Although such generalization from the interpersonal domain to the professional skill domain may be unwarranted, people do often think in this way. And, if they have no previous experience to go on, their judgment of the dentist will be based on what information is readily available to them—interpersonal behavior. To be more exact, what is most important in this situation is how the patient *perceives* the dentist and the dentist's treatment. The accuracy of the patient's perceptions is of little consequence. That is, if the patient perceives the dentist as demeaning, no matter what the dentist actually said or meant, this perception forms the basis for the patient's reaction.

In the case of Marvin, for example, we have no way of knowing whether or not his dentist actually made insulting remarks about his teeth. Marvin may be overly sensitive about his appearance and set to interpret any remark as derogatory, even if it is not meant to be so. As we will learn in later chapters, it does not matter. The truth of the matter is unknown, but the interpretation and its effect are clear.

In summary, the interpersonal behavior of the dentist is one source of fear and avoidance of dentistry. In some cases the fear may be a result of dentists' negative remarks or actions. In others it may be a result of patients' tendency to over-generalize or to make faulty interpretations. However, in either situation, the dentist must assume responsibility for positive communication and take steps to prevent misinterpretation of his or her words and behavior.

INDIRECT EXPERIENCES LEADING TO DENTAL FEAR

Many people are fearful of dentistry even though they have never had direct painful or negative experiences themselves. For example, most of our patients come to us afraid of root canal therapy. Although few have previously experienced such treatment they *know* the treatment must be painful and for them this can be a self-fulfilling prophecy. In this section we will discuss two ways in which dental fear can be acquired independently of direct negative dental experiences.

Vicarious and Informational Sources

We learn a lot by observing others and by being instructed in how to perform tasks. In fact, when we want to teach someone something, we say, "Watch me closely so you can do it too!" We have all seen children imitate their parents and other children.

We can also become emotionally aroused by observing others experience an emotion. Being around someone who is extremely happy or joyous usually gives us a good feeling. Seeing someone extremely sad or witnessing a tragic event makes us feel similarly sad. Who has not been frightened by a horror movie, even though it is an actor on the screen who is being pursued by the monster? We are not being chased, but we have come to vicariously identify with the hero or heroine and think of their experiences as though they were our own. Such sympathetic or vicarious emotional arousal is particularly strong if we know or like the person we are observing.

Dental fear can be similarly communicated. Probably the most common source of this vicarious fear development is from parents to children. Research (see Chapter 10) has shown that many fearful children have fearful parents as well (Milgrom *et al.*, 1994). By hearing parents talk of their fear or dislike of dentistry or by seeing their parents react adversely to dentistry, children can learn that "dentists are to be avoided" and they can acquire their parents' emotional reaction to the whole concept of dentistry.

In our experience, many parents are fully aware of this vicarious process. Many of our fearful patients seek treatment for their fear so that they will not pass it on to their children. Recall the example of Joan in Chapter 1. Her dental fear began when she saw her mother upset and crying at the dentist's office before she herself had ever gone. Years later when she came for treatment, her expressed reason was that she wanted to overcome her fear so she would not transmit it to her two children, as her mother had transmitted it to her.

The Mass Media

Other vehicles for communicating specific fear information are the many forms of mass media. For instance, cartoons in newspapers and magazines are full of characterizations of dentists as inflicters of torture. The cartoon shown below is one example. Just as people can communicate information, so can such pictures. The message of this cartoon is clearly spelled out: "If you go to the dentist, you can expect to be hurt." Such information, or "misinformation," can reinforce any other similar messages one may have received from parents or others. Consider the potential effect of these two sources of fear information together. Before directly experiencing dentistry, the reader of this cartoon will expect that, if and when she does go, traumatic things will occur. With this expectation, she will enter dental care with considerable anticipatory anxiety. Then, she may perceive even mildly uncomfortable stimulations as painful so her worst fears are in fact realized. Dentistry will be painful. (This relationship between being aroused and the enhanced perception of pain will be described in greater detail in Chapter 3).

Stimulus Generalization

We introduced stimulus generalization earlier in this chapter. It is the process by which a person conditioned to respond to one stimulus (CS) associated with pain or trauma will also respond emotionally to similar stimuli or situations. Through this process some people, who have never had direct negative experiences with dentistry, might respond adversely to elements of the dental situation that are reminiscent of another similar situation in which they have been traumatized. One common situation to which this applies is medical/surgical procedures. Such responses are often very perplexing to dental personnel and even to patients: it does not seem rational that just because one situation was aversive, another should be as well.

An excellent example of generalization was described by Borland (1962).

> Many years ago I did some extensive dental procedures in the mouth of a young housewife who fainted every time we began a session in the chair. This continued for a number of appointments until one day I returned a few minutes late from a luncheon club meeting to find the patient already in the chair. I went into the operating room in a business suit and injected the anesthetic, and waited for her to faint. She did not, but on the next appointment, when I was dressed in a white jacket, she fainted as reliably as ever. Subsequently, I always wore a sport shirt rather than a white jacket when treating this patient, and the fainting stopped. Discussions with the patient after the treatment was completed revealed that she had been terribly frightened when she had under-

gone a tonsillectomy as a child, and that she still had occasional nightmares about this in which the element that she
described the most vividly and with the most feeling was the
white uniforms worn by the doctors and nurses. This patient
was not reacting to me, but to a very distorted *percept* of
me—a percept whose distortion seemed to be particularly
mediated by the white uniforms. When this element was
removed from the situation, her perception of the situation
was determined more by its real characteristics and less by
the attributes of an old experience of which it reminded her.
Her feelings, from which she defended herself by fainting,
were quite appropriate for the original situation but quite
inappropriate for the contemporary one (p. 188).

This account of stimulus generalization illustrates several points
important to a full understanding of the etiology and treatment of
dental fear. First, it shows that one does *not* have to have been
harmed by, or in the presence of a dentist to react adversely to
dentistry. This reaction itself was in no way the fault of a dentist.
Second, it shows that people may have very different reactions to
fear. In this case, rather than showing the more common symptoms
associated with arousal of the sympathetic branch of the autonomic
nervous system such as increased heart rate, and respiration, the
patient appeared to show arousal of the parasympathetic branch,
resulting in a drop in heart rate and blood pressure and syncope.
Although less common among fear reactions than sympathetic
responses, this parasympathetic arousal is often seen among those
with fears of blood and injury (Connolly *et al.*, 1975). A third point is
Borland's interpretation of the patient's responding to a "distorted
percept." Rather than characterizing her reaction as *distorted*, it is
more accurate to think of this in terms of her reacting to a specific
stimulus of white coat, which was highly similar to the situation in
which she acquired this CER. We need not imply that the patient's
perceptions were in any way deviant; knowing her medical history,
the reaction is realistic. Had a full medical history been taken earlier
in which the patient could recount her experience, the dentist could
have prevented her syncope from the outset.

It is partially for reasons of stimulus generalization that many
dentists have changed the atmosphere of their offices. Rather than

sterile-looking white offices and uniforms, today we see more soft, comfortable interior decorating with carpeting, colored chairs, art work, and plants. The dentist and auxiliaries often wear colorful, patterned attire. Few stimuli remain that are clearly associated with the traditional dental and medical settings. Many fearful patients who have avoided dentistry for years comment on how these changes make them feel less threatened and more comfortable. However, these new surroundings cannot *prevent* the development of fear. Should a patient be exposed to painful or fear-eliciting stimuli in this setting, it could become a CS for fear as well.

Another common source of fear reactions to dentistry caused by stimulus generalization is an experience that virtually all children go through when they receive immunization injections. This may be one of the reasons that fear of the local anesthetic injection is so prominent, as discussed in Chapter 1. The following example illustrates this process of fear developing in one situation and generalizing to another.

> Joe was a 20-year-old college student when he was referred for fear treatment to one of us by a general practice dentist. Joe had avoided dentists for at least 10 years. When he developed a severe toothache, he got up his courage, made an appointment, and went to the referring dentist. However, when the dentist attempted the anesthetic injection, Joe jerked his arms up in front of his face and pulled his legs up to his chest. He curled up into a ball. He wasn't going to allow the injection to happen. The dentist then administered nitrous oxide and Joe appeared much more relaxed and reported that he was ready. As the syringe approached his mouth, his reaction was the same. He curled up again and would not allow the injection to happen.

When we interviewed Joe before treating him for the fear, he described where this reaction originated. As a child about age 10, he recalled standing in line at school where all the children were receiving immunizations. When he got near the front of the line, he observed the child ahead of him being injected. The child screamed and jerked, and the syringe separated from the needle, which stayed in his arm. Joe vividly recalled seeing the child crying with the needle dangling from his arm. Joe ran away and would not allow the nurse to give him his injection. As a result, he avoided dentistry altogether. As a teenager, when his mother made dental appointments for him, he conveniently "forgot" them and never went. Not only did he avoid going to the dentist, he avoided even *thinking* about going.

Joe's fear was acquired vicariously through observation; even though he was not hurt by the injection, the fear developed and generalized to all situations involving needles, including dentistry.

These two examples illustrate how fears, developed in medical settings, generalize to dentistry. Although the dentist in both cases could do nothing about the origins of these reactions, he could have identified their source by using appropriate assessment methods before treatment. He would then have been in a better position to deal with the fear reaction at an earlier stage of treatment. Dental fear has been shown to be associated with fears of heights, flying, and enclosures (Fiset *et al.*, 1989), and fearful patients may be troubled by other psychopathology, especially anxiety, mood disorders, and substance abuse (Roy-Bryne *et al.*, 1994). Techniques for assessing such problems and for treating them will be described in later chapters.

Helplessness and Lack of Control

The last two sources contributing to dental fear are related to each other and are extremely important, though somewhat less specific than those discussed thus far. Both involve more thinking and interpretation of situations by the patient. The first involves situations in which people experience a *sense* of helplessness over something that may cause them discomfort, pain, or injury. Feelings of helplessness are important in their own right as a cause of fear and intimately affect one's reactions to sources of fear. Moreover, eliminating these feelings is critical to overcoming fear.

Feelings of helplessness often accompany perceptions of lack of control. Before proceeding with our discussion of lack of control, it is important to indicate what is meant by *control*. A simple but useful definition is given by Thompson (1981), who states that control is "... the belief that one has at one's disposal a response that can influence the aversiveness of an event" (p. 89).

A critical element of this definition and the discussion to follow is the word belief. If a person believes that he has no means of influencing a negative effect, he will feel helplessness and perceive a lack of control. Extensive research has shown that such feelings and perceptions lead to fear. The opposite belief, that one *does* have control, can lead to lessened fear. This is the case whether or not the person in fact has control. It is effective so long as she believes she has control.

This effect was clearly demonstrated in a study by Geer and colleagues (1970), in which a group of subjects initially were given a series of 10 painful electric shocks. Throughout the experiment, subjects' electrodermal responses were measured as a physiological indicator of their anticipatory anxiety before each shock. They were also required to press a button immediately following each shock. They were told initially that this would be a measure of their reaction time.

After the first 10 shocks were given, half of the subjects were told that if they pressed the button quickly enough they could shorten the duration of the shock to 3 seconds. Actually, unknown to the subjects, the experimenters had arranged all shocks to be 3 seconds, but this statement created the belief that it was the subjects themselves who controlled the duration. The other half of the subjects were simply told that the remaining 10 shocks would be shorter.

During the second series of 10 shocks, the group who were led to believe that their speed of responding was responsible for the shorter shock—that is, who felt they controlled the duration— showed dramatically less physical arousal to the shocks than did those who believed they had no control. In this study, both groups received exactly the same number and duration of shocks. The only difference responsible for one group showing less anxiety was their belief (erroneous) that they could do something to influence the shock.

The study demonstrated one means of exerting control over an aversive event. There are other forms of control that also have direct relevance to dental fear and anxiety. The four types of control described by Thompson (1981) are: Behavioral, Cognitive, Informational, and Retrospective.

Behavioral Control. This category includes situations in which the person believes that he can make some behavioral response that will terminate, shorten, or lessen an aversive event. The study cited above was an example of behavioral control because the subjects believed that a rapid button press would shorten the duration of the shock. Those who were not told that they had such a response available believed they had no control and showed more fear arousal. An example often used by dentists is to tell patients they can signal him by raising their finger or hand to indicate that a procedure is becoming stressful. Again, we must emphasize that all that is necessary for this control to reduce anxiety is for a patient to *believe* that he can control the aversiveness of the event.

The feelings of lack of behavioral control are often cited by our fearful patients as either causing or contributing to their dental fear. They report that "... the dentist wouldn't stop when it hurt." "He wouldn't give me more Novocain when l asked." Such incidents would easily lead patients to believe that they have no control. In fact, the only control they believe they have is to not go to the dentist.

Cognitive Control. Cognitive control involves something that patients can do mentally to lessen the aversiveness of the stimulation or their reaction to the stimulation. Here we will focus on the lack of cognitive control, or patients' inability to control negative thoughts concerning what might happen to them while undergoing dental treatment. Fearful patients often report that both before and during dental treatment, they experience repeated negative or "catastrophizing" thoughts that keep them anxious.

In a recent study, an attempt was made to identify what fearful and non-fearful persons thought about and said to themselves while viewing a videotaped simulation of a dental restoration. People who characterized themselves, before the study, as fearful reported thinking "catastrophizing" thoughts. That is, they thought of all the possible negative or catastrophic things that could happen, such as, "What if the needle slips," "This is going to be very painful," "I can't stand it another minute," etc. Of the subjects in this study who experienced catastrophizing thoughts, 87 percent were from the high-dental-fear group. In contrast, the vast majority of those in the low-fear group reported either no specific thoughts or used coping thoughts that helped them control any anxiety, such as: "I can trust this dentist," "It's really not that bad, it could be worse." Others recalled pleasant memories, some from dentists, others from being in comfortable places. These coping thoughts provided the subjects with some cognitive control over a potentially negative situation. In contrast, catastrophizing subjects who felt they had no control, based on their thought reactions, continued to be fearful and reported that the film made them much more anxious and caused them more physiological arousal than was experienced by those who used some cognitive control strategy.

Information. The information that gives the person under stress some feeling of control includes what the situation or procedure is like, warnings that the aversive event is about to occur, and what sensations the person is likely to experience. This issue boils down to how much to tell the patient about what will transpire during treatment.

The extent to which such information or lack of it affects one's reaction to specific stimuli depends on several complex factors. We will start by discussing the simplest case: providing a warning or signal that something aversive is about to occur. Seligman (1975) contends that it is important to know when an aversive event is going to happen. When it is clear to people that they will be signaled whenever something negative will happen, this amounts to a "danger signal." Then, if it is clear that all danger will be signaled, absence of the danger signal or warning can be taken as a "safety signal." When the safety signal is present there is no need to be anxious. Therefore, the anxiety or fear arousal will be only periodic and short lasting. Being in a potentially threatening situation and never knowing when the actual negative event will occur keeps one in a continuous state of anticipatory anxiety. Lack of any information results in the patient being uncertain about what might occur. It is like a fear of the unknown. That is, the person is anxious because he does not know what the safety signals are.

Some patients report that they dislike (or fear) dentists because the dentist never told them or signaled when he would give them the local anesthetic injection. "My dentist would tell me to look the other way. Then when I looked back, he had the needle ready to stick me. He was really sneaky and I didn't like that."

Under such conditions of uncertainty, the patient knew she would receive an injection but was never sure just when. This kept her in a constant anxiety state that contributed to her overall fear of dentistry. Distrust develops in such situations.

Other information given to patients involves detailed, accurate information about the procedures that will occur and what sensations patients are likely to experience from the procedures. Presumably, if the patient does not know what is going to happen and what to expect, he will not only have anticipatory anxiety, wondering or "catastrophizing" about what might occur, but he will also be startled or surprised when it does occur. If the patient is prepared for what is to come, his fear of the unknown will be lessened and he will need to rely less on his imagination to determine what will happen. Further, once experiencing an anticipated sensation, he will know that the experience is normal, rather than something to be concerned about.

The research concerning whether or not to provide patients with information generally shows that lack of information may result in fear. However, a couple of other factors qualify this conclusion. First, the positive effects of information tend to be enhanced when the patient not only is given the information, but is also given a way of coping with any response that might result from this information (Thompson, 1981). In Chapters 6 and 8, we discuss how information and a breathing exercise were helpful for fear of anesthetic injections.

A second qualification of the effects of information on anxiety is that *some* people prefer *not* to know *what* will happen or *when*. Giving these people too much information may actually make them more fearful. Consequently, it may be useful to ask patients how much information they would like to have. Probably the majority of patients prefer to be informed, and for them, the information appears to reduce fear. Not informing them will make them fearful as it did this patient: "I am afraid of pain and the unknown. Before childbirth and before I had surgery, my doctor explained everything that was going to happen and I wasn't afraid anymore. No dentist has ever explained anything to me and I'm afraid 'cause I don't know what will happen."

Retrospective Control. This final category of control differs from control in the sense that we usually use the term. It refers to the patient's identifying the cause of an aversive event, *after* it has occurred. Once a patient can attribute the cause to something rational it gives the event more meaning and can reduce the long-term reactions to it. For example, an avoider who has been treated for his fear may become aware that anticipation, not the dental treatment itself, is his biggest problem. At this point, he is well on his way to being able to control future anticipation. For another variation on retrospective control, consider a patient who is required to undergo extensive restoration treatment that may be quite uncomfortable, painful, and anxiety provoking. If such patients identify the reason they are in this condition as their previous neglect of their oral health care, they know the responsibility lies with themselves, not the dentist nor the instruments. Further, knowing that we are personally responsible tells us what we must do in the future to prevent its recurrence. In this sense, through retrospect, the situation has meaning and order and provides a sense of control in that we know what to do to avoid or lessen future discomfort.

The Meaning of the Event

The foregoing discussion indicates that when most people are about to experience an unpleasant event, and when they believe they have no means of influencing the event, the result is fear and greater pain. A useful unifying concept to tie together the several methods of control is to consider the *meaning* that the event has for the person. If the meaning of the impending event is: "I will experience more discomfort (fear, pain, embarrassment) than I am capable of tolerating *and* I have no means of escape or control," the result is fear. Conversely, *if, in the face of threat, the patient can exercise control if desired, the meaning of the situation changes. It is more tolerable and less fear producing.*

Using this perspective, we can analyze the development of dental fear in terms of what dentistry means to patients. To begin this analysis, consider the question: "Where does meaning come from?" In brief, meaning develops out of our direct and indirect experiences with dentists and similar situations: through Conditioned Emotional Responses, dentists' personal and professional characteristics, from information communicated by friends, family, and the media. Through these experiences dentistry takes on meaning as either something positive and approachable or something negative that is to be avoided. As part of the process, we develop our beliefs about our ability to control the situation, if necessary.

If our experiences have been painful or frightening *and* we believe we have no control over them, dentistry will be something to fear and to avoid. On the other hand, if our experiences have been positive or if we feel that we can effectively control any aversiveness, then we can approach dentistry with little or no fear. For the patient whose experiences have been positive and who believes he or she is in the hands of a highly skilled and competent dentist, the issue of control becomes moot. In fact some patients report that when they are under the care of a professional who is perceived as attempting to minimize harm to them, personal control is not even preferred (Thompson, 1981). This patient says, "Do whatever is necessary—you're the doctor."

The preceding analysis then brings us back to a central issue mentioned previously: that the dentist is the most salient feature of dentistry, and it is from the dentist's behavior that much of the meaning of dentistry is derived. With this background concerning the causes of dental fear and the importance of control over aversive situations, let us now analyze the dental experiences of Harry, who before coming to our fear treatment program had avoided dentistry for eight years.

> My first recollection is having teeth pulled. I was around age 6. I was taken to the hospital and had some permanent teeth cut out or pulled out. I can still remember the mask coming down over my face and the strong smell of ether. Then I had a Technicolor dream of a train running over me which I can still remember. I remember waking and everyone being nice but being scared.
>
> Later when I was 7 or 8, the dentist didn't give me enough Novocain when filling my teeth and I cried out. He slapped his hand over my mouth hard and said "Shut up."
>
> Then about 8 years ago, I had a terrible toothache and I went to another dentist. He proceeded to pull the tooth under Novocain but the pain was excruciating. So he stopped with the tooth half out and cracked and told me to go to an oral surgeon. I can still remember the pain while waiting to have that tooth cut out.

Several points from Harry's history with dentistry illustrate the concepts discussed earlier. Harry's first experience with dentistry at age six was very frightening. He had no control over what was happening, and even though he did not recall any specific pain, his perception of what happened was that he had teeth *cut* out, a frightening thought to a young child. Although the people were "being nice," he was still scared. Dentistry now had some meaning to him.

His next experience involved pain at the hands of the dentist. Not only did he have no control, he believed that he was abused by the dentist for attempting to control the situation. The meaning of dentistry was clearer to him by then.

Finally, his last appointment involved severe pain and no opportunity to control it. The pain was extended by his having to wait for the oral surgeon to complete the extraction. Harry had all of the conditions for the development of dental fear: fear of the unknown, extensive and extended pain, perceived abuse and unprofessional behavior by the dentist, and no means by which he could control either his or the dentist's reactions or behavior. By this time, dentistry had a very clear meaning to Harry.

A MODEL OF DENTAL FEAR ACQUISITION

In the preceding sections we described the various processes that contribute to a patient's fear development. In this section we integrate these processes into a comprehensive model. This model will serve as a basis for guiding our discussion throughout this text and points to methods for preventing and treating dental fear. As can be seen in the schematic presentation of the Model in Table 2-1, the two major factors involved in fear development are: (1) the patients' earlier experiences with dentistry, direct and indirect, and (2) the patients' perceptions of whether or not they have or could have control over what will happen to them if they wish it. Each of the four combinations will be discussed in turn.

TABLE 2-1
A Model of Dental Fear

Dental Experiences	Patient Perceived Control	
	Yes	*No*
Positive	—no fear	—no fear
	—approach	—approach
	—highly positive attitudes	—highly positive attitudes
Negative	—Some anticipatory anxiety possible	—fear
	—no or little fear	—avoidance
	—mostly approach	—highly negative attitude
	—attitude highly positive to mildly negative	—highly negative attitude

Positive Experiences and Perceived Control

As suggested in the previous sections, patients whose experiences with dentistry have been positive and who have been led to believe they can control any negative or painful stimulation are unlikely to experience dental fear. They will not avoid dentistry, and their general attitudes toward dentists and dentistry as a profession will be highly positive. Factors contributing to this positive outlook on dentistry would likely involve early encouragement and positive communication by parents; actual dental experiences of a positive, relatively unpainful nature; and services from a dentist and staff who communicate to the patient that she is seen as a unique individual who will be treated with respect and who will have, if desired, some say in treatment. The result would be a satisfied patient who is unlikely to miss appointments *and* a patient who is cooperative and a pleasure to treat.

Positive Experiences and No Perceived Control

Patients falling into this category may be very similar to their counterparts with positive experiences and control. They are not likely to experience fear so they probably will not avoid dentists in the future. Given their positive experiences, the issue of control becomes less relevant. Recall in our previous discussion of research on perceived control that some people who believe they are in the care of a competent and trustworthy practitioner may actually prefer to relinquish control. In either case, whether or not they actually prefer to leave control in the hands of the provider, the fact that they have little or no need to control the situation renders the control issue moot.

Negative Experiences and Perceived Control

Those patients who have had some of the negative experiences noted previously but who do believe that they have control, present a more mixed picture. Here we need to describe several alternatives encompassed in these conditions. For many in this group, there is likely to be at least some level of anxiety. The extent of the anxiety would largely be determined by the number and intensity of their past experiences. If a patient has had several negative experiences at the hands of a dentist other than the one who currently provides the sense of control, the patient would likely experience some anxiety. This might last until he or she was able to actually experience some measure of control. In fact, we have found that approximately one-fourth of low-fear patients who describe early painful experiences have changed to dentists with whom they feel more comfortable (Bernstein *et al.*, 1979).

Another variation involves patients who have had to undergo extensive restoration and describe the experience as very painful, but who do not develop fear as a result. The surveys discussed earlier indicate that some non-fearful patients described early painful dental experiences. Approximately 40 percent of these patients also made complimentary comments about their dentists. We interpret this to mean that it is not necessarily painful experiences themselves that cause fear. Rather, in the presence of pain, the factor that determines whether or not fear will result is how the dentist deals with the patient's pain. As one low-fear patient from our survey described her experiences, "Dr. Rosen was great. Whenever it would hurt, he would stop until I felt better before starting again." Pain experienced by a patient in control is not likely to lead to fear.

It is the interaction of the dentist and the patient which determines whether fear will result from pain.

Negative Experiences and No Perceived Control

With these two conditions present, we feel that fear is almost an automatic outcome. The patient who has been led to believe that dentistry is painful, whose actual experience is traumatic, and who has no feeling of control over the situation will develop fear, avoid dentistry, and have negative attitudes toward the profession. From the dentist's point of view, when and if such patients appear, they will be difficult to treat and stressful for dental personnel. However, we wrote this book precisely to facilitate treatment of this group. It is our belief and experience, supported by research, that the fear can be treated and that fearful persons can be introduced into the ranks of satisfied, cooperative, and enjoyable patients.

A MODEL OF DENTAL FEAR TREATMENT

To complement the preceding model of dental fear development, we now introduce a model of dental fear treatment. This model is essentially the converse of the fear development model and will serve as the basis for the several treatment approaches to be described in detail in Chapters 5–9.

The model derives from a cognitive, social learning approach to fear reduction, as described by Albert Bandura (1977). It is cognitive because an important element in identifying and changing dental fear behavior is how the person *thinks* about himself in the feared situation. It involves social learning because a patient learns new ways of thinking and behaving (e.g., fearlessness). And this learning takes place in a social context involving information acquired from others, especially dental personnel. Dentistry is as much a social situation involving interaction with others as it is a technical process.

In its basic form, this model proposes that fear and avoidance behavior are acquired through a variety of direct and indirect experiences. These experiences and their effect on the patient's perceptions of dentistry leave the patient with certain *expectations* about what will occur. If the expectation is that "I will experience pain and humiliation, and be unable to control myself or the situation," anxiety, fear, and avoidance will result. In other words, if a patient's past experience has led him to believe that what he will encounter at the dental office is beyond his coping ability, he will experience fear.

Given this conceptualization of fear development, the focus of treatment is to change patients' expectations about what they will experience and their ability to cope with what they do experience. This is often referred to as enhancing a patient's sense of *self-efficacy*.

The model also proposes various means for changing these expectations so the person can enter or re-enter dentistry and feel more confident of his ability to cope. Here, we will briefly outline the types of experiences that can contribute to changes in their beliefs or expectations. To parallel our fear development model, we can separate these into direct and indirect experiences. Then we add a third category of experience: learning coping skills. As we will see, several types of experiences often need to be combined in order to most effectively change one's expectations and fear. An outline of this fear treatment model is shown in Table 2-2.

TABLE 2-2
Outline of the Treatment Model:
Sources of Expectancy Change and Fear Reduction

Direct Experiences
1. Patient exposed to non-traumatic dental treatment
2. Patient experiences sense of control if desired

Indirect Experience
1. Patient observes others undergoing non-traumatic dental experiences (live or on video)
2. Patient receives information on modern dental treatment

Development of Coping Skills
1. Learning to relax in dental treatment
2. Learning to pace and breathe deeply
3. Learning positive self-statements
4. Avoiding negative "catastrophizing" statements
5. Learning to distract self
6. Learning to talk to dental personnel to exercise control if needed

---

Sources of Expectancy Change

Direct Experiences. The most reliable and most powerful means of reducing fear and changing one's expectancy about dentistry is to have direct positive experiences. In the same way that direct negative experiences create fear and negative expectations, direct positive experiences show the patient that what he will experience will run counter to his expectations of trauma. This actual exposure to dentistry without negative consequences serves to alter his future expectancy of trauma and thus begins to extinguish conditioned emotional reactions.

As with any other learning process, complete change may take several exposures to be fully effective. Further, since fearful patients hold negative expectations, they may initially feel unable to cope with a full treatment appointment. Consequently, dental personnel may need to structure short initial appointments with minimal treatment. As patients experience success in coping with each stage, they expect to be better able to handle later stages, and their fear decreases. Chapter 4 contains a discussion about planning dental treatment to provide short positive experiences. Enhancing control (and trust) is an important part of providing new and positive experiences. Chapter 5 presents specific strategies to enhance trust and control.

Indirect Experiences. Indirect experiences which communicate to the patient that her negative expectancies are exaggerated can also contribute to fear reduction. Vicarious experiences, such as observing others undergoing non-traumatic and positive dental treatment, can serve this purpose. Such modeling procedures have been widely and successfully used, especially with children (Melamed *et al.*, 1978; Williams *et al.*, 1983). Other indirect exposures that change expectancies include reading about "modern dentistry," seeing film strips describing what actually occurs, and simply talking to others who have had positive experiences with trustworthy dentists. Although these latter procedures are unlikely by themselves to eliminate fear entirely, they may provide sufficient change in expectancy to allow the fearful patient to take the first step toward direct exposure.

Learning Coping Skills. The final category of treatment procedures to change fear is aimed directly at enhancing patients' perception of their own abilities to cope with dentistry. Included are techniques for learning relaxation skills to be applied before and during treatment; training in making coping and positive self-statements to replace negative catastrophizing statements; distraction procedures; and training in talking to dental personnel to facilitate patients' feelings of personal control over what is happening to them. These skills are discussed in Chapters 6–9.

In general, this model proposes a variety of procedures aimed at changing the patients' perceptions of and experiences with dentistry. In most cases, it may be necessary to combine several of these procedures for successful fear treatment. The indirect experiences and training in coping skills may be necessary to bring the patient to the point where he is ready to directly experience non-traumatic dentistry. We believe that it is through this direct exposure to dentistry, conducted by observant, trustworthy, and concerned dental personnel, that significant change occurs in patients' expectations and fear.

SUMMARY

In this chapter we have outlined the major processes by which patients develop their fear and avoidance of dentistry. We showed that direct experiences with painful or frightening dental situations could lead to *conditioned emotional responses* in which the dentist or some aspect of dentistry became associated with the trauma. Through these experiences, elements of the dental situation acquired the capacity to automatically elicit an emotional response, even without the original unconditioned stimulus being experienced.

Another source of direct experience leading to fear concerned the *dentist's behavior* toward the patient. Such dentist behaviors as belittlement, scolding, or an impersonal, uncaring attitude also contribute to patients' fear and lack of trust. Further, we noted that the critical element was not just how the dentist behaved, but how the patient *perceived* or interpreted what the dentist did or said.

Some people appear to be fearful of dentistry even though they themselves have had no direct negative experiences. For these people, we discussed several types of indirect experiences that contribute to fear. These include *vicarious experiences* and receiving *information* communicated by others, which led patients to believe that dentistry could harm them. Similarly, we noted the abundance of *mass media* with jokes and cartoons depicting the horrors of dentistry.

Other patients who have never directly experienced dental trauma may have acquired their fear of dentistry through *stimulus generalization.* Such patients may have experienced fear or pain in other medical settings, and because of the settings' similarity with dentistry, the original reaction can be elicited by the dental situation.

Important in its own right and contributing to the other sources of dental fear are the patient's feelings of *helplessness* and *perceived lack of control* over potentially threatening situations. Four types of patient control were mentioned and the effects of their absence were described: *behavioral control, cognitive control, informational control,* and *retrospective control.* The sense of control that a patient felt or did not feel contributed to the *meaning* that the situation or event had for him. If the dental situation meant to the patient that he or she would experience discomfort and have no means to control or escape it, the result would be heightened anxiety or fear.

We described a *model of dental fear acquisition* that combined patients' experiences with the notions of perceived control. We noted that when negative experiences were present *and* the patient felt no sense of control, fear was the likely outcome.

Finally, we presented a model of dental fear treatment that focused on changing patients' *expectations* concerning what might occur at a dental office. We noted that we could most effectively counter these expectations of trauma by gradually providing patients with direct positive dental experiences in which they are given a sense of control, both over the procedures being conducted and over their own reactions to those procedures.

QUESTIONS AND EXERCISES

1. Recall the last time you had any medical or dental treatment. What were the salient features of that appointment? What things did you like and what did you dislike about the facility or provider?

2. Talk with six dental patients or friends who have expressed being fearful of dentistry. How closely do their accounts or stories mesh with those described in this chapter? Were they basically the same or were there other causes?

3. From you discussion with the six individuals, identify the unconditioned stimuli and identify statements that pointed to helplessness and control issues.

4. What is the difference between being at a horror movie in which you experience vicarious fear and a situation in which you believe you may actually be injured? One dimension of difference is that you know one is real and one is not. What other similarities and differences are there in these two situations?

5. Specify the differences between the four types of control.

THREE

The Assessment Process in the Office

- Recognizing Anxiety
- The Initial Examination
- Health Professional Hesitancies in Talking to Patients about Their Fears
- The Emergency Examination

In the preceding chapter, we discussed conceptual models to explain the processes underlying fear and pain. These models provide a framework for understanding clinical problems. Now we will focus on applying these concepts to assess dental fear.

The first step is to conduct a thorough examination of the problem. This may occur in a variety of ways. For example, in order to determine the status of a particular tooth you may utilize an explorer, periodontal probe, X-rays, and vitality tester. The process of evaluating the psychological state of a patient is no different from the diagnostic process used for determining the health status of a tooth; only the tools differ.

Thus, in working with the fearful patient, the dental procedure does not change; you simply have an additional set of data: the patients' fears. With the very fearful patient, this may be the crucial factor determining whether you are successful with a patient.

Anxiety is generally referred to by laymen as though it connotes a specific set of feelings and behaviors. Although such usage is common, it belies the complexity of the concept. It is critical to realize that the labels *anxiety* and *fear* are general concepts for a variety of feelings and behaviors. Recall that anxiety is a response in anticipation of a dreaded event, while fear is the response in the presence of the stressor. Both problems are discussed in this and the following chapters.

Some patients may have an overriding fear of pain, while others will report a fear of feeling totally helpless or claustrophobic. It is crucial to understand that fears and anxieties may differ from one patient to another although they all have a common theme of dental fear. It is also important to realize that people express signs of fear in three different areas: *the patient's behavior*—what we see the patient do—such as gripping the chair arms tightly; *the patient's physiological responses*—such as rapid breathing or profuse sweating; and *the patient's self-report*—what the patient says about his fear. When taken together, signs from these three areas indicate the presence of a constellation of emotions we label as fear or anxiety. It may be expressed in any one of these areas alone or in combination. For example, a patient may report feeling terrified and yet appear calm and physiologically unaroused while in the chair.

You can identify the fearful patient at three points: after treatment has begun, during the initial appointment, and before the initial visit. Obviously, the earlier you are able to determine that the patient is fearful, the greater the probability of your success in working with her. Consequently, we will first examine how you can identify and then work with the new fearful patient.

In keeping with what we have said about expressions of fear, there are three primary sources of information for making an assessment: *self-report* (what the patient tells you), *behavioral signs*, and *physiological indicators*. Signs in any one or a combination of these systems may indicate the presence of fear. But any one sign, taken by itself, tells us little without other information. Confounding the problem of identifying anxiety is that responses in these three areas do not always occur simultaneously (Rachman & Hodgson, 1974). They may show *desynchrony* or not be in "synch" with each other. For instance, a person might deny or not admit that he is particularly fearful, yet show significant physiological changes when seated in the operatory. This is particularly true when fear levels are moderate. Similarly, a patient might come yearly for an examination, behave like a model patient, yet report being terrified. To complicate things further, different patients respond with different physiological signs when they are upset. For example, one patient might break out in sweat but show relatively little change in heart rate, while another might have quite the opposite pattern. On the other hand, some patients may deny having elevated levels of anxiety while showing physiologic or behavioral signs of anxiety equal to or greater than responses found in high-anxiety patients. While reporting low anxiety, such patients (Weinberger *et al.*, 1979) have been found not to cope very well in the dental environment (Fox *et al.*, 1989). We have found that some of these patients are concerned about the safety of the anesthetics or other drugs or procedures, as they are aware of physiological arousal, yet others deny dental fear while tightly clenching their fists or tensing other muscle groups. Needless to say, such people may be difficult to treat in a routine and straightforward manner.

This lack of strict correspondence among and within the various systems that indicate fear can lead to erroneous assumptions concerning the patient's actual psychological state. Overall, we believe that it is usually best to trust the patient's self-report, even though this sometimes runs counter to our sense and instruments. We will now examine the three ways of assessing anxiety in more detail.

RECOGNIZING ANXIETY

Self Report

The patient serves as a primary source of information. However, such information cannot always be taken at face value because the conditions under which it is obtained can influence its content and validity. Most patients are embarrassed about their fears and are very sensitive to appearing silly or are afraid of being belittled. If the patient feels uncomfortable talking with you, he may say nothing about, or minimize, his fears. We find that most patients must be encouraged to talk about their fears.

Self-reports concerning fear of dentistry can be obtained at the time of the initial telephone contact, or through an assessment interview, or questionnaires. We will first examine the opportunities for identification when the patient initially contacts the office. In Chapter 4 we will examine the assessment of fear through the use of interviews and questionnaires.

Initial Contact. The best time to identify the fearful patient is *before* a visit, during the initial telephone contact. If you add a few questions to the information the receptionist normally obtains before the first appointment, you can identify many fearful patients. Here are questions that might be included in the initial telephone intake.

1. How long has it been since your last dental visit?

2. What kind of treatment did you have? How was it? How did it feel?

3. Do you have any concerns about receiving dental treatment that would be helpful for us to know?

Question 1: How long has it been since your last dental visit? That is, why did the patient decide to make an appointment at this time rather than six months ago or six months in the future? Patients often report they have called because "A filling fell out a few months ago, I've been having a dull ache for a week," or "I've been putting it off for years and I know I have lots of problems, so I finally forced myself to call, or, "I called because my spouse asked me to."

Fear, being too busy, and finances are the three reasons most often given for not seeing a dentist in three or more years. Fearful patients often wait until they think something is wrong. These "reasons" should alert you to explore further if you hope to make this new patient into one who returns regularly. For example, if the patient had no money before, what has changed? Or if the patient avoided because of fear, what can you do to help the person overcome their fears so that he or she will return once the emergency is solved? Less common is the patient who has recently been to another dentist, but was "dissatisfied" or had a traumatic experience with that dentist.

Question 2: What kind of treatment did you have? How was it? How did you feel? It is important to remember that you are seeking the patient's perception of the experience, how he remembers it. You may know (or think you do) that his report is exaggerated or could not be accurate. That is unimportant at this point. Your task is not to try and correct a patient's misunderstandings or to doubt the experience. Instead, it is to understand how the patient perceives the experience.

Question 3: Do you have any concerns or difficulties about receiving dental work that would be helpful for us to know? This question can "open the door" for a patient to talk about how she feels.

Alternatively, you may have your receptionist make some kind of statement to each person seeking an appointment, such as: "I don't know if you are aware of this, but our dentist has a special interest in working with people who are apprehensive about dental treatment. How have you felt about going to the dentist?"

For those offices which routinely provide a packet of materials for the first-time patient to complete before the initial visit, we recommend using the Corah Dental Anxiety Scale. One of the most widely used and researched, it is short and easy to complete. As you can see in Figure 3-1, its primary focus is on the anticipation of dental treatment. The research indicates that it is highly correlated with observed and reported dental anxiety (Corah, 1969).

Many people, of course, even though not particularly fearful, report that they do not enjoy going to the dentist. Screening questions help you identify those people who find dentistry truly aversive and are willing to admit it. Identifying such patients before their first appointment allows you to structure their dental experience differently from that of the regular patient.

CORAH DENTAL ANXIETY SCALE

1. If you had to go to the dentist tomorrow, how would you feel about it?
   a. I would look forward to it as a reasonably enjoyable experience.
   b. I wouldn't care one way or the other.
   c. I would be a little uneasy about it.
   d. I would be afraid that it would be unpleasant and painful.
   e. I would be very frightened of what the dentist might do.

2. When you are waiting in the dentist's office for your turn in the chair, how do you feel?
   a. Relaxed.
   b. A little uneasy.
   c. Tense.
   d. Anxious.
   e. So anxious that I sometimes break out in a sweat or almost feel physically sick.

3. When you are in the dentist's chair waiting while he gets his drill ready to begin working on your teeth, how do you feel? (Same alternatives as number 2.)

4. You are in the dentist's chair to have your teeth cleaned. While you are waiting and the dentist is getting out the instruments which he will use to scrape your teeth around the gums, how do you feel? (Same alternatives as number 2.)

Points were assigned for the subject's choices, with one point for an (a) choice to 5 points for an (e) choice.

From Corah. N.L. Assessment of a dental anxiety scale, *Journal of Dental Research*, 43:406, July–August 1969. Reprinted with permission.

FIGURE 3-1. Corah Dental Anxiety Scale.

If a patient is identified as being fearful before his first office visit, what should you do? Thank the patient for sharing that information and reinforce him for taking the first step of making an appointment. Let him know that the dentist will want to learn more

about his concerns in order to figure out haw to make him as comfortable as possible. We recommend that some "extra" time be set
aside in the dentist's schedule to establish rapport and explore the
patient's worries in more detail.

Before examining the use of other self-report techniques in the
initial appointment and during treatment, we will review the
behavioral and physiological signs of anxiety, which can be observed
when the patient first comes to your office.

Behavioral Signs

The patient's behavior in the waiting room can provide an early
indication of whether or not she is anxious. However, like other
types of information, waiting room behavior by itself can be considered only as a possible sign of anxiety. Nonetheless, there are data
suggesting that fearful patients display more movement in the
waiting room than do non-fearful patients (Barash, 1974; Kleinknecht
& Bernstein, 1978). In particular, fearful patients frequently display
more arm and hand movements than non-fearful patients, rapidly
thumbing through magazines and fidgeting with their hands or
other objects.

Because the receptionist is in the most advantageous position to
observe patients in the waiting room, she could make a note to cue
the other staff members to explore the issue further before beginning
the dental examination or treatment. And if the earlier phone
interview revealed that the patient had not been to a dentist for
several years, or had problems with other dentists, behavioral
observation could help to confirm dental fear.

Figure 3-2 is a checklist of behavioral signs of anxiety that the
receptionist might observe in the waiting room.

If the receptionist is included in the fear assessment team, it may
be helpful for her to fill out a form, such as the one in Figure 3-2,
and give it to the first clinician scheduled to see the patient. Once
again, however, we caution against making premature judgments
based only on waiting room behavior. Patients may be active and
anxious for reasons other than impending dentistry. For example,
they might have experienced a near auto accident on their way to the
office or they might be concerned about being late for another
appointment. Moreover, some displays of anger are very similar to

anxious behavior and may or may not be related to dental fear.

BEHAVIOR CHECKLIST

Pt. Name   ____   fidgeting with hands or objects

_____   ____   sitting on edge of chair leaning forward

                    ____   rapidly thumbing through magazines

Date   ____   pacing

_____   ____   changing sitting position frequently

                    ____   startled reactions to ordinary office noises

                    ____   rapid head movement

                    ____   repetitious hand/leg and foot movement

                    ____   other

FIGURE 3-2. Checklist To Be Used By Receptionist.

Interestingly, in Chapter 1 we reported a study showing that specific behaviors associated with fear in the operatory take essentially the opposite pattern from what occurred in the waiting room. That is, high-fear patients moved less, talked to the dentist or assistant less, and held their hands clasped more than low-fear patients. Further, the behaviors that most clearly differentiate high- from low-fear patients occur before actual treatment when the patient is alone in the operatory or when either the dentist or the assistant is present but not yet involved in treatment.

Observation of patient behavior in the operatory gives you the opportunity to further test out a hypothesis and to discuss observations with the patient either at that time, or if more privacy and detailed discussion appear warranted, during a more extensive interview.

Physiological Signs

Activation of the autonomic nervous system (ANS) under stress provides another constellation of fear indicators. Under ideal conditions, changes in organ systems enervated by the ANS can be precisely monitored with a polygraph. Unfortunately, such instrumentation is both too cumbersome and expensive for routine use in a dental office. However, signs of ANS activation are readily observable.

There are three physiological indicators that can readily be observed in the office. One of the most clearly observable signs is excessive perspiration. Those areas particularly sensitive to "arousal sweating" (Kuno, 1956) include the palms of the hands, underarms, forehead, and upper portions of the lip. The latter two are observable, the former easily assessed by a handshake.

The second set of signs are the cardiovascular responses. They include pulse rate and blood pressure. For patients whose fears focus around catastrophic physical reactions, we frequently utilize a portable heart rate monitor to give them feedback. Pulsation in the carotid and temporal arteries can also be observed from the dentist's typical working position. Observation of arterial pulsation has the advantage of being unobtrusive and the dentist can do it periodically to assess changes throughout an appointment.

Finally, observation of the depth and rate of respiration can provide yet another index of anxiety. Rapid, shallow breathing suggests increased arousal. Similarly, a patient's *holding* his breath is a common sign of fear. This is most likely to occur during a procedure in which the patient fears he may be hurt—for instance, in the injection or during extraction. These observations may be most effectively made by the assistant while the dentist is involved in the treatment procedures

THE INITIAL EXAMINATION

From a dental standpoint, the purposes of the initial exam are to obtain an accurate picture of the patient's overall dental health and to reach a tentative diagnosis. From a patient management perspective, the exam has three primary functions:

1. To present information in a positive manner in order to mitigate the patient's fear of receiving "bad news."

2. To let patients know that they will be consulted and listened to regarding treatment preferences.

3. To demonstrate to patients that they will not be surprised or be

"forced" to do anything against their will.

It is important to remember that during the initial examination your words and gestures are being scrutinized very closely. At this point patients try to determine if you are really different from other dentists and dental personnel they have known. Because the dental environment is so familiar to us, we forget that to many patients dentistry is mysterious or threatening. Consequently, the overall rule is to inform the patient what it is you wish to do, what the purpose is, and ask if it is "OK" to proceed.

It is important to conduct procedures in order of priority. The longer the exam process, the greater the anxiety most fearful patients will experience. Thus, proceed to gather only the most essential information: the condition of carious or damaged teeth or periodontal condition of key areas of the mouth. Reserve the "nice-to-know" aspects of the exam, such as periodontal probings of all the teeth or the condition of asymptomatic third molars, for another visit. These data may be important but are best gathered after you have established more rapport with the patient. Painful tests, such as electric vitality testing, can be carried out after you review radiographs. For many highly fearful patients, your initial exam may have to be conducted visually without the explorer or periodontal probe. Only when trust is established can you gain permission to use these other instruments. Avoid using air syringes or water with these patients. If the teeth are covered in plaque, use a wet 2x2 cotton gauze and gently wipe the teeth. Your gentleness will be appreciated by the prospective patient.

It is easy in the interest of "thoroughness" or simply habit to push the patient beyond the point of her comfort. It is important to remember that your primary goals at this point are to demonstrate to the patient that she has a say in what happens and to have her return. Initially, the patient has few effective skills for coping with dentistry. Consequently, until the patient is taught how to cope differently, it is the health professional who must modify what he or she does. Otherwise, the dental experience will most likely be a repeat of past negative experiences with the same consequences, which is most often a disappearing patient.

Vocabulary is also important. The patient will usually not understand technical vocabulary and may be frightened by certain other terms (e.g., root canal). At the same time, he may perceive pedodontic terms (e.g., "putting the tooth to sleep") as patronizing and they may breed distrust. Our experience is that you should use lay terms as much as possible and avoid detailed explanations. To the extent that explanations are necessary, there will be time for them later, after a therapeutic relationship is established. It is important to remember that fear, like any other intense emotion, impedes our ability to hear a message. We still hear the words, but

HERMAN®

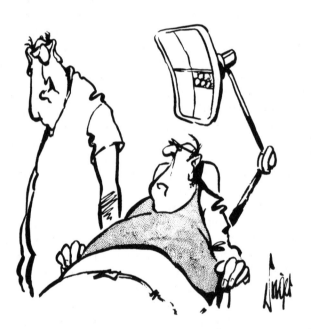

**"Why don't you have a good scream and
get it over with."**

our "perceptual filters" change and selectively screen out parts of the message. In the Dental Fears Research Clinic, we routinely begin the examination by trying to explain what we are doing. Imagine the following conversation:

> Dentist: I want to take a thorough look at your teeth and gums to learn about what's going on in there. To do that I want to use my mirror and explorer. Is that OK with you?
>
> Patient: Yeah, but don't stick that pick in my teeth!
>
> Dentist: O.K. I will be careful. While I do this I will ask Jane, my assistant, to write down information, so that I can make a map of your mouth. Most of what I will say will be about work that has already been done--in other words it won't all be bad news! After I'm done I will explain to you in "English" what I find and you can ask questions. Are you ready to begin?

Such an explanation helps to reduce the patient's fears. It lets him know that a time to talk and ask questions will follow the exam. We encourage patients who are obviously fearful to bring a friend or significant other to the office and to accompany them into the operatory for the exam. The friend may be able to "listen better" than the anxious person, and frequently acts as a strong supporter afterwards in encouraging the patient to proceed with treatment.

Asking Permission

You will note in the previous conversation that the dentist asked twice if what he proposed was "OK" with the patient. We do not ask these questions rhetorically. Using this technique allows you to accomplish two patient management objectives: letting the patient know that he will be consulted, and informing him that there will be "no surprises." Your asking permission allows the patient to feel that he has a role in treatment. Frequently patients feel that they do not know what is going on, and that they have no right to participate or comment about their preferences for treatment. The importance of this is clear when you consider how people act when they are afraid. Fear makes a person hesitant to "go ahead" with the frightening event. Thus, a patient who feels he is "being pushed" may find a way to resist. We have met many patients who failed to return to other dentists for treatment after being "frightened to death" about the work needed. Or having returned, they refused to begin treatment. Similarly, many practitioners have expressed their frustration about spending hour-long appointments without success trying to persuade a patient to proceed, without success.

Asking permission places the responsibility for treatment with the patient. You may question: "Don't patients abuse this privilege? Who's in charge here, me or the patient?" Recall that one of the most common fears is of being helpless and under the control of the dentist. We have all been taught to check during treatment with a patient, "How are you doing?" In the same way, asking permission is checking to see if the patient is ready to proceed. It enhances the patient's control, and has the paradoxical effect of allowing progress to be made more quickly than if you tried to push the patient.

Concluding the Initial Examination

At this point you should explain your tentative conclusions. Because of our professional training, most of us begin by listing the most severe or emergent problems we have found. For example, a dentist might begin by saying:

> "The primary problem is this tooth that hurts. It looks like you will need a root canal, which is a procedure where we take out the nerve and replace it with an inert plug. You have two new cavities that need to be filled, and a few old fillings that should be replaced. You also have moderate periodontal disease which will require treatment. This may sound like a lot of work, but it is all pretty routine dentistry, and everything should turn out 'OK' by the time we finish."

What is wrong with this approach? First, it focuses exclusively on problems. Second, it begins by mentioning the need for a root canal, one of the most feared procedures in dentistry. With this beginning, the probability has increased dramatically that your patient will not remember half of what you have said and will not return. Also, for some patients, the implied cost (psychic and financial) may be overwhelming.

As we discussed in Chapter 1, Gale (1972) reported that the third most common fear mentioned by patients was of "hearing bad news." Our clinical experience supports this finding. At times fears are very specific: "I know the dentist will find all my teeth have to be extracted," or "All my expensive crowns are failing." Clearly the examination appointment will be stressful for these patients. Other patients, though not fearing a specific calamity, are convinced—usually because they have not seen the dentist in a few years—that "the doctor will find something horribly wrong with me." Their imaginations run wild during a routine exam. Imagining that every-thing written down is "another problem," such patients can become so anxious that by the time you are ready to explain what you have found, they cannot listen to what you have to say.

Compare the previous summary with the following:

> "Let me begin by saying that most of your teeth are in good shape. You have two kinds of problems, and both can be successfully treated. I'm glad you came in now, rather than waiting longer. We can make you healthy again. The first, which I am most concerned about, is the infection in your gums. It is the infection which makes your teeth so sensitive, and the condition which can eventually cause more problems than anything else.
>
> The second problem involves your teeth. There are two new cavities and three old fillings that need to be repaired. All of them involve routine work and the teeth will be 'good as new' after we're done. The last tooth I want to discuss is the one that you pointed out as bothering you. Although I need to do some more tests, it looks as though that tooth will need more complicated treatment, which I will explain in detail later. It too should turn out fine. I want to give you some antibiotics to reduce the infection in that tooth (which also will help the gums). Also, I'd like to start with some simpler procedures so that I can get to know how you react to treatment, and you have a chance to get to know me. Do you have any questions?"

In summary, your task is to let the patient know what is "OK" about his health, and present the problems in a non-overwhelming way so that the patient can understand that there is a solution.

History Taking

Medical Conditions Influencing Fear Treatment

It is beyond the scope of a textbook on fear to comprehensively review medical history taking. Today, diseases of the immune and endocrine systems and habits like smoking are taking on increasing importance as we treat dental patients. For those who need a refresher, we recommend a text such as *Internal Medicine for Dentistry* by Rose and Kaye (1983). Nevertheless, there are some special considerations worth your attention in talking with the fearful patient (Milgrom & Weinstein, 1993).

In study at the Dental Fears Research Clinic we found that the majority of fearful patients had periods in their lives when they abused alcohol or other drugs. (Roy-Bryne et al., 1994). Relatively few active drug users or alcoholics seek treatment. And although the proportion of patients with a substance abuse history will not be as high in a community practice, it is important to learn about this history because it may predict pain control problems during future treatment. Many of these patients will tell you that they have had experiences of poor pain control in the past. The problem is not unique to dentistry and occurs in anesthesiology practice in the hospital as well. We do not know exactly why this problem occurs and the sources are under study at our clinic. The problem may stem from altered physiology, cross-tolerance, or expectation. Nevertheless, being forewarned allows us to alter our anesthetic regime if necessary (Fiset et al., 1989). Similar problems with post-operative pain control can be expected. In addition Milgrom et al. (1993) found that patients with a past or present history of substance abuse may not improve as much as patients with other psychiatric diagnoses. Questions you could ask include, "How much alcohol do you drink each week?" "Have you ever had a period in your life where you have problems with alcohol or drugs?"

A related history topic is the patient's experience with local anesthetics or other medications. If a patient reports a sensitivity to local anesthetic or presents you with a request to use anesthetic without vasoconstrictor, you should take a careful history (Fiset *et al.*, 1990). Try to elicit the detailed circumstance surrounding previous experience. Refrain from making any judgments about the problem until you can request records from previous providers. Talking with previous dentists often will allow you to make a differential diagnosis between true sensitivity, previous overdose or intravascular injection, or just anxiety over injections resulting in physiological upset. Some of these patients will require allergy testing to rule out allergies. This problem is discussed further in the section on patients who are afraid of medical catastrophe. Nonetheless, the key to managing these types of problems is to take them seriously and not to adopt unusual treatment strategies, such as eliminating the vasoconstrictor from anesthetics, unless you really understand the problem and its history. Acting on limited knowledge merely reinforces the patient's misunderstanding of the previous experience and makes it harder for him to receive care.

There has been much in the professional literature lately about latex glove allergies. Because of possible untoward hypersensitivity responses and true allergy, we routinely question Dental Fears Research Clinic patients about their experiences in this area. The literature suggests that most of the problems are confined to those people, such as health care workers, who use gloves routinely. Nevertheless, we treated a patient who developed facial erythema and edema every time she had a dental visit where gloves were used or a rubber dam was placed. After treatment for anxiety, the symptoms disappeared (Longley *et al.*, 1993). Patients who report adverse effects to local anesthetics and other dental materials are discussed in more detail in Chapter 8.

Medication histories are also very important in treating fearful patients. They can tip you off to an underlying anxiety problem. Patients who are chronically taking benzodiazepines may have pain control problems at the dentist. Patients on low dose tricyclics may be receiving treatment for chronic facial pain. Often patients are unaware of exactly why they are taking some medications.

Consulting with Physicians

At the Dental Fears Research Clinic we routinely request written releases from patients to obtain medical records and consultation. This allows us to fully understand a patient's history before talking with the physician. For example, a patient reported to us that she experienced anaphylaxis in an emergency room after being given a local anesthetic. A review of the emergency room record showed syncope was the problem. Another patient reported that she was afraid of dying from a reaction to dental drugs because her heart was weak. She had recently moved to town and could not find a physician who would take her concern seriously. After our evaluation, we were able to help find a physician who was willing to request the records from another state. It turned out that the patient had an underlying anxiety disorder that had been misdiagnosed. With proper medical and psychological care the patient was able to receive routine dental treatment.

When calling a physician, always give the receptionist the name of the patient and suggest that the chart be pulled before you speak to the doctor. Ask if it would be better if he or she called you back after looking over the record. Advise the physician that you are treating a dentally anxious patient. If you are requesting allergy testing, tell the physician that you will be sending several articles from the literature about the problem that he or she may find useful. Often it is helpful to ask the physician to make a note in the chart about your conversation or for you to follow-up with a letter confirming your discussion or specific request for evaluation. For a more detailed discussion on making referrals see Chapter 8.

Health professionals' hesitancies about talking to patients about fear

Interestingly, research has shown that while most dental health professionals feel that they can easily recognize the anxious patient, most attempt to do little about the problem. Corah and colleagues (1985) found that two-thirds of the dentists they surveyed tend to avoid doing anything about the patient's fear if they feel that the patient will be cooperative. Thus, most practitioners try to be kind and gentle in the hope that the patient can make it through treatment. Further, nearly 80 percent of the dentists reported that they themselves were anxious when working with anxious patients. It was also found that dental professionals hesitate to talk directly to patients about fear because they are concerned that they may make the problem worse.

To complicate the picture further, it is extremely common for a fearful patient to make every effort to "be a grown up" and co-operate. However, there are problems associated with trying to gloss over the fear. Almost every patient can force herself to get through any procedure on any given day. For example, it is almost always possible to "snag" the pulp of an infected tooth. However, as any experienced clinician knows, this does not mean that the patient will return for the "easy" appointment of having the canals obturated. Your goal is to have the patient return.

We believe that fear should be put on the problem list just as is cardiovascular disease or diabetes. It is a problem which will affect the course of treatment. We believe that the health professional should raise the issue directly. The patient needs to know that you consider such problems a part of "normal" practice and that you have some knowledge about how solve them. The situation is analogous to that of a swimming or skiing coach. He is not supposed to be a psychologist, but he must recognize that some of his students are hesitant and anxious. He must find ways of working with them to ensure that they have a positive experience. Otherwise, they too will not come back.

As you will learn, the treatment of simple fears and phobias is relatively straightforward and well within the skill level of the interested, trained practitioner. However, there are other psychological problems which interfere with dental treatment, but which are too difficult for the average practitioner to work with successfully. The purpose of this section is to help you recognize and screen such patients, rather than to tell you how to treat them.

Recently 73 consecutive adult patients at the Dental Fears Research Clinic at the University of Washington were systematically evaluated via a structured psychiatric interview and standardized questionnaires (Roy-Byrne *et al.*, 1994). Results indicate that 40 percent of people seeking treatment for dental fear had major psychiatric diagnoses in addition to simple dental fear. These diagnoses were primarily anxiety or mood disorders. Similar findings have been suggested by Israeli scientists (Kleinhauz *et al.*, 1992).

Questions about worry/anxiousness and fear of other situations are crucial in helping you determine the nature and scope of the patient's fears. For example, "Do you find any other situations as difficult (scary) as going to the dentist? Are you taking any medications for psychological conditions? Do you consider yourself to be a nervous/high strung person? How do you feel about medical care such as blood draws or innoculations?"

Questions about trust and competence are also important. Distrust, like every human emotion or condition, comes in all degrees of severity. Sometimes it is very specific to dentists, or health care professionals. However, there are other situations when the distrust you detect is part of the individual's *overall* view of life, and is not specific to certain situations. Such distrust is considered in the psychiatric classification system as a personality disorder. When the distrust is so pervasive, it will often be almost impossible to establish a successful working relationship. Questions that you might ask include: "Have you had any bad experience with dentists or physicians where you felt that they were incompetent or did not have your best interests at heart?" "Do you consider yourself a pretty trusting person overall, or much more the skeptic?"

To summarize: the practical question the dental health care professional faces is, "How big a problem or barrier to successful completion of the proposed treatment is the patient's psychological attitudes and beliefs?" A general rule of thumb is this: Assessment is the key. Chapter 4 will discuss the assessment process in detail. In the case of psychological problems the task is to determine how narrow (or widespread) the problem appears to be in the patient's life. As a general rule, the more areas in which the person appears to function normally; the more able he is to cope with the strains and stress of modern life; the less "disturbed" he is; and the easier it will be for you to work with him successfully. Conversely, the more situations in which he has problems, or appears unable to cope, the more difficult the task will be.

What should you do when faced with a patient with significant psychological problems? If the patient is already in psychotherapy or counseling, we suggest that you ask permission to contact his or her therapist. Some people may need to address their larger psychological issues before they are ready to tolerate dental care: in these situations a referral is appropriate. See Chapter 8.

Caveat. Many people have gone through difficult times in their lives. Many of us have had periods when we abused drugs, or have been severely depressed; or we have had panic attacks associated with a particularly stressful event, such as getting divorced, losing a job, etc. However, it has been our experience that if those problems are in the past, especially if the person sought some type of help for them, it is unlikely that they will act as barriers to treatment. Similarly, if the person has some current problems but is under the active care of a physician or psychologist, it is likely that the problems will present only minimal barriers. However, if you determine that the person has a number of coping problems which have not been addressed, or are not being treated, it will be much more difficult to work with him. To use an analogy, if a person is being treated for blood pressure or diabetic problems, it is possible to work with her as a dental patient. However, if the medical problem is not being managed it is unwise to commence dental treatment. So too with obvious psychological problems. Sometimes the best thing that you can do is make a referral to an appropriate mental health counselor.

THE EMERGENCY EXAMINATION

Because so many fearful patients are first seen on an emergency basis, it is important to consider what we can do in order to help him break the pattern of only seeking symptomatic care and turn him into a regular patient. Chronic avoiders frequently have badly broken-down teeth and acute endodontic and periodontic lesions. Pain will bring them to the office, and provides an opportunity to break the chain of symptomatic treatment.

Several general rules are helpful. First, be available. Return emergency telephone calls promptly and do not delay scheduling appointments. Second, use the first few minutes to establish rapport. Only if the patient sees you (and your staff) as non-judgmental and truly supportive will he return. Expect to see problems and try to see this visit as an opportunity to bring a reluctant patient to the benefits of good oral health, however slowly. Finally, try to use pain medications and antibiotics, if appropriate, to get over the acute phase.

If at all possible, avoid operative or surgical treatment at the time the patient is in pain. Any dentistry at this point will probably hurt the patient. Training in dental schools often creates the impression that every abscessed tooth or hyperemic pulp is a dental emergency requiring drainage or pulp extirpation. A true emergency is a situation with fever, extensive swelling, or patient dehydration. In most cases, however, operative intervention can be delayed. It can be argued that endodontic treatment or surgery in these situations, is correct medically. On the other hand, it disrupts your practice and too often results in liability claims because of mistakes made during the disorder of an ill-planned emergency treatment that could have been avoided.

Our goal is to help the patient break out of his seeking treatment only when he is in pain. A review of emergency records in most clinics reveals that patients who are offered immediate treatment usually do not return. Thus, from a behavioral point of view, this treatment is ineffective. After the painful episode is over, you and your patient can create a treatment plan that addresses fears and provides the positive experiences that are required to overcome the avoidance that has resulted in the emergency episode in the first place.

Suggested Procedure

Take the following steps. First, assess the situation and decide if a true emergency exists. State your goal that you want to avoid providing painful treatment and that you want to have them return. Discuss what has stood in the way of the patient seeking care in the past. Talk in terms of lowering the barriers to care that the patient perceives rather than emphasizing the benefits of good oral health. The former approach creates an opportunity for the patient to return while the latter usually just causes embarrassment. In our experience, most fearful patients already understand that dentistry is beneficial, if only they could tolerate it. Second, provide reassurance and explain the nature of the problem simply. Be sure the patient knows how to get in touch with you after hours in case things go sour. Emphasize your availability.

Third, prescribe the medications required. Most patients with toothaches know what medications are effective for them and we are often surprised when patients tell us that Extra-Strength Excedrin™ (aspirin/acetaminophen/caffeine) or Tylenol™ (acetaminophen or paracetamol) is their drug of choice. On the other hand, if the pain is acute and the patient can tolerate aspirin-like drugs, we prefer Ibuprofen, 400 mg every three to four hours. Is it as effective for dental pain as the codeine combinations, which are not available in many countries outside the U.S., and does not cause as much nausea. Ibuprofen is widely available 24 hours a day without prescription in many countries.

Do not hesitate to prescribe narcotic analgesic combinations such as acetaminophen (500 mg), paracetamol-codeine (30 mg), similar aspirin combinations, or hydrocodone (5 mg)-acetaminophen (500 mg) if the patient has had good experience previously. Caution against taking too much drug on an empty stomach because the resultant nausea can be worse than the pain. While you may be concerned about "professional" patients seeking drugs, the risk is relatively minor when the quantities prescribed are small. In the Dental Fears Research Clinic we do not generally prescribe oxycodone (Percodan™) based drugs. These drugs have greater potential for abuse; more importantly, they cause a lot of nausea and they are not particularly superior in pain control to the other drugs described earlier. Our view is that pain control for the patient is the primary concern. Most pain of the type we are describing is moderated by these drugs and runs its course within 24 to 48 hours. If patients are still seeking medication after that, other strategies may be needed.

Many authors advocate the use of long-acting anesthetics injected (e.g., 1.8-3.0 mL bupivacaine 0.5% with 1:200,000 epinephrine) to provide up to 12 hours of relief for pulpitis (Moore and Dunsky, 1983). Our experience is that this combined with analgesics can provide enough relief for the patient to sleep and calm down. The problem is that many fearful patients avoid injections and few will willingly accept this approach. Moreover, the length of pulpal anesthesia with these drugs is very much shorter; thus, the effect of the soft tissue anesthesia may not be worth all the negatives associated with trying to inject anesthetic in a "moving target."

The effects of antibiotics are slower and less predictable, especially for inflamed pulps. Nonetheless, we recommend use of the penicillins or cephalosporins for pulpitis or acute periodontal abscesses. Consider one week, 500 mg four times per day after a loading dose of 1000 mg. Monitor the patient carefully. If a fever or acute swelling develops, see the patient immediately and seek specialty consultation if in doubt about any aspect of the case.

Finally, schedule a follow-up visit within one week. At that visit start the process of a thorough examination of the dental condition and the fear. Out of pain and grateful for your concern, most fearful patients will be receptive to beginning treatment.

Emergency Endodontics

The strategy outlined above takes care of the vast majority of emergency situations. However, if after 24–36 hours the pain does not abate, you may need to go ahead and open a tooth or debride a periodontal abscess to establish drainage. Be sure to do a careful differential diagnosis before you begin. Fearful patients will report colorful symptoms. They may report sinus or muscle pain as unbearable tooth pain and, the unwary clinician may prescribe unnecessary endodontics or surgical treatment for the patient.

Schedule enough time. Do everything you can not to traumatize the patient. First, do not give long, scary explanations. Keep it simple. If the patient has not had any pain medication within four hours, dispense Ibuprofen (400 mg) or acetaminophen (500 mg) preoperatively. Second, use lots of anesthetic. Stick with the anesthetic you usually use and anesthetize a larger than normal area. In the mandible, inferior alveolar blocks require at least 3 ml of Lidocaine 2% with vasoconstrictor and probably more. If possible, use a vitality tester to assess anesthesia and supplement the initial injections with septal or ligamentary injections until you are successful. Try to eliminate as much pain as possible. If the patient is fairly calm, we teach basic breathing skills right away and then try to introduce nitrous oxide. The purpose of using nitrous oxide in this situation is pain, not anxiety, control. It is delivered at a high volume at 50% nitrous oxide – 50% oxygen and is usually necessary only during the injection and initial drilling.

Third, use careful technique. A preoperative radiograph and rubber dam are mandatory. Use a new bur. When drilling, structure time. Tell the patient that you will drill for a count of one. Stop after a second and ask the patient how he or she is doing. Then proceed again, with a count of one or two. Breaking the drilling up allows the patient some control over the situation, and if it hurts, most can get through it successfully. Avoid the temptation to just get it over with. This exacerbates the patient's loss of control and discomfort.

After the initial pulp extirpation, allow frequent rest breaks—every few minutes ask the patient to sit up and sip some fruit juice. Be supportive and let the patient know everything will turn out OK. Try not to appear rushed and avoid anger and put-downs if the patient has trouble with the visit. Finally, try to fully instrument the tooth at this time; endodontic research suggests that this is the best way to avoid recurrence of pain. Be sure the patient has adequate pain medication and urge him or her to take the medication preventively for the next 24 hours regardless of whether or not it hurts at the time.

After the treatment is finished, we always debrief the patient. "How did it go?" "Could I have done anything to make it easier?" This is a good time to provide reassurance and laud the fearful patient for doing well under adverse circumstances, whether or not there were tears or upset during the procedure. Fearful patients are often very tough on themselves out of worry about the disruption they are causing you. Check with this patient by telephone frequently during the next several days to make sure the patient is comfortable and to double check that he is taking pain medication correctly. For more discussion on pain control, see Chapter 7.

SUMMARY

In this chapter we have examined the importance of openly and directly discussing the patient's fears of dental treatment. Assessment of the patient's fears is best begun as early as possible. Behavioral signs, physiological signs, and self-report are the three primary sources of information for making an assessment. The initial appointment is a critical period in the treatment of a fearful patient. In order to get a patient to return, you must work to appear nonjudgemental about their dental condition and accepting of their fears. Because the patient's skills at coping with treatment are presently not very effective, it is up to the health professional to modify early treatment to make it tolerable.

We discussed some basic principles of emergency treatment, as so many fearful patients appear in the office for the first time because of acute pain. Delaying invasive procedures when possible increases the probability the patient will return.

Finally, we attempted to put the problem of fear into perspective by discussing patients who have more significant psychological problems. In the next chapter we will discuss in detail how to go about assessing the nature of the patient's fear. This will provide the basis of selecting specific treatment strategies which are discussed in the remaining chapters.

QUESTIONS AND EXERCISES

1. What are the reasons why it is important for dental health professionals to assess a patient's fears?

2. What is the importance of trying to assess anxiety in more than one way? Explain desynchrony.

3. What is the suggested method for handling a fearful emergency patient? How does this strategy differ from how you might treat a non-fearful patient or one who has been a part of your practice for years?

4. What specific steps can you take to reduce patient anxiety during the initial examination?

FOUR

Psychological Assessment of Fear

- Diagnostic Categories of Fear
- Diagnostic Categories versus Psychiatric Diagnoses
- Assessment Measures
- Treatment Planning

UNIVERSITY OF WASHINGTON DIAGNOSTIC CATEGORIES OF DENTAL FEAR

We present here a helpful diagnostic approach that groups patient fears into four types and we discuss management techniques appropriate to each specific type of fear. A diagnosis is useful only if it leads to differing treatment strategies. By the same token, a skilled clinician will consider many factors when planning complex treatment, such as a complicated restoration. Knowing that there may be a number of possible solutions to the problem, the practitioner may weigh the patient's concern with esthetics, health care habits, financial resources, and gingival health before deciding on an appropriate treatment strategy to recommend. A somewhat less skilled clinician, however, may attempt to treat similar technical problems the same way each time he sees them, based on a fixed ideal of "the way it was taught in school," or of a personal philosophy of "I do only first-class 'Cadillac' restorative work." Each of us has probably seen examples of technically excellent dental work where the plan was nevertheless inappropriate for the particular patient. This discussion holds true for the treatment of dental fear, where there is no single approach or technique that works equally well with every patient.

This classification system attempts to bring order to a complex area of behavior. The specific clinical strategies suggested in later chapters are based on these diagnostic categories. The categories were developed out of our work with patients and they have proved clinically useful in treatment. Note that these categories are neither psychiatric nor psychological diagnostic classifications and are not intended as such. Our purpose is not to turn the dental reader into a psychologist but to provide a framework for understanding the differences between patients. We will discuss how standard psychiatric diagnoses relate to this system at a later point.

As we examine the four diagnostic categories of fear, it is useful to think of each category having as its root a specific kind of fear. However, we must also emphasize that people (and their fears) do not always come in neat packages. A person may exhibit fears from more than one category but, as we described in Chapter 2, the feeling of lack of control in the dental situation is a theme common to all types.

The first category is the *fear of specific stimuli*. It is based on a fear of being unable to tolerate a particular procedure, or the pain the patient associates with dental treatment. The second is *distrust* of the dental provider. This category may include one or more of the following: a loss of self-esteem as a result of perceived belittlement; a feeling of helplessness and victimization in the dental situation; or suspicion and doubt of what the dentist says or does. All reflect communication failures. Third is the category we call *generalized anxiety*. Patients in this category find many different situations to be difficult and stressful. They tend to habitually worry and believe that they cannot adequately control or manage their own upsetting thoughts. The final category is the *fear of a medically overwhelming catastrophe*. It is based on a fear of having an uncontrollable bodily reaction to dental treatment, such as a heart attack, choking, or an allergic reaction.

As we discuss each category in more detail, we will review composite descriptions of patients who represent each of the four categories of fear. The descriptions are, so far as possible, in the patients' own words so that we can give you a clinical picture showing how these patients appear in the dental office. The descriptions are organized into the composite patients' dental histories, presenting complaint, feelings about control, medical history, and social-psychological status. How to elicit relevant diagnostic information is discussed following the descriptions.

Category 1: Fear of Specific Stimuli

Dental History. Patients can usually state clearly what aspect of dental treatment is aversive to them. "I can't stand needles." "The pain of the drill is the worst part." "Fillings are fine, I'm just terrified of having a tooth pulled." "If it didn't hurt I would be fine." The patient's problem appears specific and focused, while he sees other aspects of treatment as tolerable.

Note: Patients often mention pain and the fear of feeling pain when asked why they fear dental treatment. This is the "expected" answer, and pain is frequently a *contributing* factor. However, it is important to assess whether pain is the *predominant* fear or is secondary to other concerns such as worry or distrust. When it *is* of primary concern, patients are emphatic that it is the pain they fear and they can usually trace the origin of their fears to specific experiences: "When I was 14 years old, the dentist pulled my tooth without me being numb." The fear of pain is focused around a very specific agent such as the needle or drilling. Such patients often avoid dental care for very long periods.

Presenting Complaint. "I hate dentistry (nothing personal). I have a low pain tolerance. I don't mind anything except the pain of that drill." "The dentist would tell me it wouldn't hurt, but it always did." "I have a difficult time getting numb." "I'd rather go with a toothache than go through that drill." "I just hate needles."

Control. Patients fear they will have no way to prevent the aversiveness of the experience. "I had horrible experiences with drilling as a kid. My dentist never used enough Novocain. I told him it hurt and he just kept on going." "You might as well be strapped down once the dentist begins to work."

Medical History. Within normal limits. Some patients report difficulties with similar medical procedures, such as injections and blood drawing if they have a needle phobia.

Social/Psychological History. "I can't think of anything else I'm afraid of besides dentistry (the drill)." "I really don't understand why I'm so fearful." "I'm a competent person, but somehow I can't talk myself out of being afraid." Patients within this category express fear, but seldom get upset emotionally with anticipation or worry in advance of the actual fear stimulus. See Chapter 8 for appropriate treatment strategies.

Category 2: Distrust of Dental Personnel

Dental History. These patients are hypersensitive to the behavior of dental personnel. They often feel, "My dentist didn't care about me," or "The dental hygienist acted like she wished I could drop my teeth off at the door in the morning," or "The billing accountant tried to pull a fast one." They often mention being made to feel guilty, or being put down for their home oral care: "I *know* my teeth are terrible, I don't need anyone to make me feel worse," or "The dentist took my fears personally and got angry because I was afraid. He told me to 'Stop acting like a baby,' or to 'Grow up'" or "He didn't let me ask questions and I never knew what was going on."

These patients are concerned with loss of self-esteem, feeling "one down," and an inability to interact meaningfully with health professionals. They have a *low* level of trust and are cynical about reassurances that "everything will be O.K."

Presenting Complaint. "I want to be treated as a person. It's important to me that I am able to communicate." "He treated me just like another set of teeth." "My dentist would become impatient when I asked questions." I never felt like I knew what was going on." "They always criticized the way I brushed my teeth. I really felt put down."

Control. Patients in this category feel that dental personnel are authoritarian and will do whatever they wish, no matter what the patient says or does. They describe themselves as feeling like victims, at the whim or mercy of the dentist. This attitude is frequently a result of repeated negative childhood experiences with a particular individual. They like information, facts, and options. They want to participate in treatment decisions.

Medical History. Within normal limits. There may also be distrust of medical personnel .

Social/psychological history. "I think of myself as being a 'rational, real world' person. I like information and read as much as possible about something before I decide about what I want to do." Many appear to be cynical, skeptical, or angry. They tend to resent what they perceive as attempts to persuade or pressure them into decisions. Some patients will appear sensitive to being taken advantage of in a variety of life circumstances. See Chapter 5 for further discussion on the treatment of the distrustful patient.

Category 3: Generalized Anxiety

Dental History. One's first impression is that this patient doesn't cope with life very well. He perceives many situations as stressful. "I have gone in to get my teeth cleaned and X-rayed, but when they told me about the work that was needed I never went back." "I've always hated going, but it's getting worse." "I make appointments and then don't go (or cancel) at the last minute. I'm a wreck for a week before my appointment."

Dental fear may be predominant, but it is frequently only one of several fears or phobias felt by these people. The most common are flying, heights, and closed spaces. Claustrophobia and the fear of being leaned back in the chair are not uncommon. When asked to describe what is so frightening about dental care, this group of patients frequently responds, "I don't know." If questioned, they often mention not sleeping well the night before the visit. This is the most common type of dental fear patient.

HERMAN®

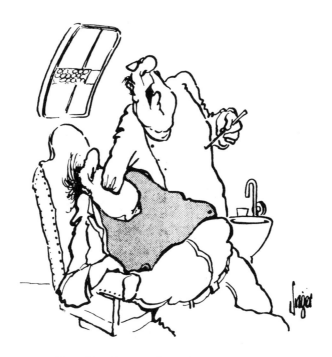

"Hold still! I dropped my little mirror."

Presenting Complaint. "Everything about dentistry is awful." "I worry about my teeth all the time. I've always had problems with my teeth." "It's a nightmare." "I can't stop thinking about it." These patients are easily overwhelmed by information, or by what appears to them to be a big dental problem. "I know I have a ton of work that needs to be done." "I don't know what to do." "I avoid thinking about dentistry; it's too upsetting."

Control. Patients within this category believe that their *thoughts* are not controllable and perceive them as "just happening." They say things like, "My thoughts run away on their own." "I can't stop thinking/worrying about it." They see events and situations as beyond their personal control because of their own perceived inadequacies. They know that *other* people can deal with the dental situation; it is their own abilities they doubt. They often are glad to hand control over to others whom they see as more competent. Consequently they are seldom information oriented and are often very receptive to suggestion and to anti-anxiety agents.

Medical History. The patient is likely to have a long history of diffuse complaints, such as stress, headaches, or digestive problems. He may report a history of "panic attacks" or depression. This group of patients is most likely to have taken various anti-anxiety medications, such as Prozac® or Elavil®.

Social/Psychological History. Most of these patients will typically acknowledge, "I'm a worrier. I get anxious about the future. ... I tend to anticipate and ruminate about problems. I'm high strung." "I have trouble falling asleep at night because my mind is so busy. There are a lot of stressful things happening in my life. I cry easily. I get depressed fairly often. I'm not very assertive. When I have a problem I wind up sticking my head in the sand and hope it will go away." Easily overwhelmed, they will frequently choose to do nothing if care is not taken to make their problems seem manageable. See Chapter 6 for further discussion of coping and cognitive strategies.

Category 4: Fear of Catastrophe

Dental History. Patients whose fears fall within this category report being afraid of experiencing a life-threatening medical emergency during dental treatment. They are hypervigilant about bodily sensations: heart palpitations, numbness of their extremities, profuse sweating, or chills. In extreme cases they may fear dying in the chair from a heart attack or cerebral aneurysm. Patients who report that they are allergic to the anesthetic, that it causes their heart to beat uncontrollably, or that it causes them difficulty in breathing, also fall within this category. "I've had a lot of dental work done, but a few years ago I began to have these terrible physical reactions to dental treatment which got worse and worse until I finally stopped going. One of my attacks was so bad I had to leave in the middle of the appointment. ... The dentist sent me home after I fainted in the chair and had me go see a physician!" "I got very panicky. ... I felt like I couldn't breathe. I had to get out of there ... I was embarrassed." Finally, there are some patients who believe that the dentist will make a critical error resulting in a medical emergency.

Presenting Complaint. "I think I'm allergic to the anesthetic. ... I'm not afraid of dentistry; I'm afraid of having an attack." "I feel like I might gag or choke to death. I have had severe allergies all my life. The last dentist told me it was all in my head because allergies are so rare. I told him I was *the* one and walked out! No one will believe me."

Control. Almost without exception, patients in this group feel that these bodily responses are beyond their volitional control. They frequently have a history of "attacks," or "reactions" and are afraid their body will "run amok." They fear fainting, not being able to breathe, or choking to death. Patients who attribute their reactions to a physical stimulus or physiological reaction will frequently state they are not afraid of dentistry, only of their involuntary bodily response.

Medical History. "I saw a physician about my problem and he suggested that the epinephrine be taken out of the anesthetic. Do you have another drug you could use?" Common physical "reactions" include: rapid heart rate, hyperventilation, numbness and tingling of the extremities, perceived difficulty in breathing, choking, gagging, and gasping for air. Patients may have a history of consulting various medical specialists about the problem or of reporting allergic reactions to a wide variety of substances.

Social/Psychological History. Patients will frequently be able to talk quite rationally about their problem. The patient's history will generally appear within normal limits except for this one area. However, probing about the patient's life activities may reveal that he restricts himself from certain situations or activities that he feels might also trigger such attacks. See Chapter 8 for a more detailed discussion on the assessment and treatment of these concerns.

Prioritizing Patient Concerns

We have presented the four patterns of fear as "pure" types for the purposes of illustration. However, people and problems seldom come in neat packages. While you will see patients who clearly fit into one category, others will appear to have characteristics of two or more categories. This leads us to ask which cluster of concerns is primary and should be addressed first, and what combinations are most common. Experience with patients over the past 14 years has taught us that, in general, whenever a patient expresses strong distrust of the dental staff it must be tackled first. If the patient has doubts regarding their competence or professional ethics, or feels that he has not been listened to in the past, this is always the primary issue. If it is not dealt with at the outset, the chances are great that your relationship with the patient will also turn sour. Similarly, if a patient is fearful of a medical catastrophe (i.e., dying), focusing on his restorative needs, or reassurances that such events are "rare" does little to address his concerns. Steps must be taken to "get to the bottom" of those worries before proceeding further. A common combination of patterns is seen in the patient with catastrophic fears and distrust. It is frequently a result of the patient's feeling that no one has taken his problems seriously. Catastrophe patients may also exhibit many signs of the generalized anxiety patient, but tend to attribute such symptoms to a malfunctioning physiology and *not* to their emotional states. Interestingly, once you help them get over their fears of an iatrogenic problem, they are usually best treated with strategies appropriate for the generalized anxiety patient.

Patients who are fearful of aversive stimuli, especially pain, may also be perceived as somewhat distrustful because have been hurt in the past by an uncaring professional. If the distrust focused, the distrust is usually of secondary concern and easily dealt with. If, on the other hand, distrust and skepticism appear to be more integral parts of the patient's personality, the specific fear (fear of the needle) is often secondary. Patients with a number of specific fears, only some of which are dentally related, often are best thought of as generalized anxiety patients.

Generalized anxiety patients seldom show signs of distrust. While they may have many intense bodily reactions, such as panic attacks, they usually recognize their thoughts and emotions as being the causes or triggers. When you determine that the patient's thoughts and emotions across a variety of situations get him into a "mental mess," where anticipation and worry create "mountains out of molehills," management of this problem must take precedence over concerns about his not being able to tolerate certain aspects of treatment. Less frequent are patients who who are both distrustful *and* worriers.

University of Washington
Diagnostic Categories versus Psychiatric Diagnoses

We have now discussed a clinical model of four different patterns, or clusters, of fears which we observe in patients fearful of dental treatment, and how they most commonly combine with each other. It is intended to help the dental professional better understand the basic nature of a patient's fears, and to guide him in choosing appropriate strategies to help the patient learn how to tolerate care. However, as noted earlier, this model is not intended to correlate with the formal diagnostic system of the American Psychiatric Association, although there is some overlap with it.

The work of Roy-Byrne *et al.* (1994) supports our clinical observations that dental phobia is a diagnostically heterogeneous category. That is, fearful patients are not all alike, and patient fears vary widely, which is why we believe that different management strategies are more effective in addressing certain types of fears. Most patients who have difficulty receiving dental care can be classified, from a psychiatric standpoint, to have one or more Anxiety Disorders (*Diagnostic Statistical Manual*, IV, 1994). These range from Specific Phobia, to others, such as Panic Disorder with Agoraphobia, which could be thought of as falling at the other end of the anxiety spectrum. A Specific Phobia is characterized by clinically significant anxiety provoked by exposure to a specific feared object or situation, often leading to avoidant behavior. Generalized Anxiety Disorder is a more diffuse problem which affects an individual's overall functioning and characteristic ways of coping, which are unrelated to any one situation. While anxiety disorders can be extremely severe and crippling, the good news is that they are amenable to change through psychological intervention techniques known as cognitive-behavioral therapy. Significant, measurable progress for even the most severe anxiety disorders can often be made within six months with the help of a competent therapist. Specific phobias, on the other hand, may often be resolved in two to four hours of treatment. Patients whom we classify as having fear of medical catastrophe are often complicated to treat. In the psychiatric system they may be diagnosed as having a Somatoform Disorder.

Mood Disorders, such as Major Depressive Disorders or Bipolar Disorders, while relatively common in the general population, are seen infrequently in the dental setting unless the patient is under active psychological treatment. Untreated individuals seldom have the energy to attend to "elective" activities such as dental treatment. Similarly, patients with active Substance Related Disorders are seldom candidates for anything but symptomatic treatment. Finally, as mentioned earlier, patients whom we classify as distrustful may range from the merely skeptical, to those with a Paranoid Personality Disorder. Deciding when and how to make a referral to a mental health specialist is discussed in Chapter 8.

As we discussed previously, there are three sources of information to determine if a patient is anxious: behavioral signs, physiological signs, and self report—what the patient tells you. We will now examine in detail various self report measures which can be used to assess a patient's anxiety and help you determine what treatment strategies to employ to help overcome the patient's fears.

ASSESSMENT MEASURES:

I.   THE STRUCTURED FEAR ASSESSMENT INTERVIEW

General Considerations

In many dental practices it is customary to automatically schedule non-emergency patients for a hygienist appointment and radiographs before the initial examination by the dentist. For the "regular" dental patient or "goers but haters," this may prove satisfactory. However, for the fearful patient this approach will frequently cause problems. A patient who has a fear of bad news, for example, may work himself into such an anxious state by the time you are ready to make a case presentation that he will be unable to attend to what you actually say. A distrustful but non-assertive patient may feel that she is getting the runaround by being seen only by auxiliary personnel.

Although it may appear at first glance to be a somewhat unusual suggestion, our experience has led us to conclude that patients whom you consider fearful should be interviewed by the dentist or hygienist before *any* treatment, including an examination. The initial relationship established will, more than any other factor, determine if the patient will enter treatment and ultimately remain in your practice. Preferably, this interview should be held outside the operatory in a consultation room. In offices where this is not possible, we recommend that the patient be allowed to sit upright in the chair and that an atmosphere of privacy be established, so far as possible. The interview could be conducted by the hygienist or dentist. Who does the interview is less important than how it is conducted.

Remember, many patients are somewhat reluctant to admit they are fearful. They have frequently received the message from friends or other dentists that they should stop being childish and "learn how to control themselves." Consequently, the more private the interview setting, the more comfortable and open your prospective patient is likely to be.

Caveat. No matter what you are doing, whenever you reach a point suspecting that a patient is fearful, it is important to quickly but gently check out your observations. You may simply report what you see. "You seem to be grasping the chair very tightly," or "You seem to be holding your breath when I work." Alternatively, inquire directly about how the patient is feeling, "Are you feeling a little nervous about the appointment today?" If a patient responds in a way to confirm your observations, it is time to lay down your dental instruments, sit the patient up, and begin talking and listening! It doesn't matter if you are scheduled to do an MO on #28. Your purpose changes from completing a dental procedure to ensuring that the patient has a non-traumatic experience.

Introducing the Interview

What can you say to the patient about your desire to talk with him regarding his "feelings about the dentist?" Imagine the following conversation:

Dentist: John, from some of the things you have said, it seems that you are somewhat anxious about having dental work done.

John: Well, yes, but then I guess everybody is a little nervous about it.

Dentist: True, but some people get more anxious than others, and before I devise a treatment plan or begin work, I would like to take a few minutes to ask you some questions. Your answers will help me know how to make your experience here as comfortable as I can. Is that OK with you?

John: Sure, why not?

Dentist: OK, good. I want to emphasize that a lot of patients are anxious about some aspects of dental care. My purpose is first to try to figure out what **I** can do to make treatment as easy and comfortable for you as possible. Second, I want to see if I can figure out what **you** might do for yourself to feel more comfortable with treatment.

It is critical before or near the beginning of the interview to convey to the patient that you take her worries and concerns seriously. That is, you recognize they are legitimate, real, and "normal." In talking with a patient you may consider the patient's fears *exaggerated*. After all, operative dentistry is familiar to you, and you know how safe, painless, and easy it can be. However, "objective facts," or what *you* know, have little influence on another person's fears. To make this clear, we often use an analogy involving some other activity. For example, we might say to the patient, "I am sure you have heard about or know someone who is terrified of flying, or swimming, or skiing. Although he knows *other* people can do it easily enough, it does not make him brave enough to try. If someone is going to learn how to do something difficult, like swimming, when one is afraid, initially, it is very helpful to break it up into small steps or lessons so as not to get overwhelmed. Dentistry is similar. It's *natural* to feel some apprehension about it. It *is* a little scary to be on your back, with people leaning over you and doing things you don't really understand, some of which are uncomfortable." The key point is to have the patient understand that you accept his fear nonjudgmentally and that you can work with him to help him overcome it.

Figure 4-1 lists the objectives of a fear assessment interview.

---

1. To visibly demonstrate to the patient that you are concerned to find out who he is, and what his concerns are.
2. To begin establishing a relationship of trust based upon two-way communication.
3. To let the patient know that you take seriously his worries/ concerns and consider them "normal."
4. To obtain the patient's point of view or perspective on the nature and extent of his fears regarding treatment.
5. To obtain sufficient information to assess or diagnose the nature and type of fear exhibited by the patient.
6. To obtain a sense of the patient's dental I.Q.—his understanding of his current problems and knowledge of dental disease and prevention.
7. To gain an understanding of how the patient copes with stressful situations.

FIGURE 4-1. Objectives of a Fear Assessment Interview

Figure 4-2 lists a series of questions that are useful in an initial assessment interview. Obviously, not every question will be asked of every new patient. However, the questions will help you obtain the information you need to assess the patient. We will discuss each question in turn, will look at typical responses, and will see how they differentiate between the four different types of fear.

Question 1: Why did you make an appointment at this time? Do you need dental treatment now?

Question 2: a. When was your last dental visit? What did you have done? How did you feel?

b. Describe your last restorative appointment (date work was performed, etc.)

1. Why did you make an appointment at this time? Do you need dental treatment now?

2. a. When was your last dental visit? What did you have done? How did you feel?

   b. Describe your last restorative appointment (date work performed, etc.).

3. In general, what are the most difficult/fearful things about dentistry?

4. What kinds of things, besides dentistry, are you afraid of?

5. How do you cope with other stressful situations?

6. What kinds of things could be done to make receiving care easier?

7. How do you feel about medical care? Blood draws? Shots?

8. How do you feel the night/morning before you are scheduled to come in for an appointment?

9. How likely are you to delay making an appointment because of your feelings about dentistry? Or to cancel it after it is made?

10. How do you feel about the idea of taking a drug to reduce your anxiety?

11. How do you feel about the appearance of your teeth? Explain.

12. In the last two years, has the condition of your teeth caused you to cancel social activities or miss work? If yes, how much?

13. Have you ever seriously considered having all your teeth pulled and getting dentures? Explain.

14. Are your friends or family aware of your fears? If so, what kinds of things have they said?

FIGURE 4-2. Structured Interview

You will recognize questions 1 and 2 as those we recommended your receptionist ask in the initial telephone intake (Chapter 3). Even if they have been asked of the patient previously, the questions provide a good starting point. They also allow you to hear in the patient's own words why he made an appointment to seek treatment at this time. By asking, "Why now, instead of six months ago," you have an opportunity to understand the importance the patient places on dental care and her feelings about it.

Questions one and two allow you to explore a factor that frequently appears to be a primary concern and is the basis of many patients' fears—the "fear of bad news." Have you ever had a series of headaches and thought "brain tumor," or persistent abdominal troubles and feared intestinal cancer, and yet found yourself reluctant to have a thorough examination? The fear of "finding out that it's really serious," and "they all have to be pulled," or that the sensitivity means "my teeth are full of cavities" contributes to avoidance of care. People who express a fear of the magnitude of a problem and a desire to avoid knowing typify those individuals falling within the generalized anxiety category.

Question 3: In general, what are the most difficult/fearful things about dentistry?

As we discussed earlier, most patients, with some very obvious exceptions, will first mention a fear of pain. This is the expected response, and it is tempting to accept these initial statements at face value. It seems logical that pain would be the most fearful aspect of receiving dental care. However, with some skillful interviewing you will find that for many patients this is only one of several issues. Thus, the task is to determine if fear of pain is primary, or only a contributing factor. Bernstein *et al.* (1979) found that over 50 percent of one sample of fearful patients cited "dentists' personal behavior and professional characteristics" as contributing to their fear of dentistry. Follow-up questions such as, "Besides the pain, is there anything else about the dental experience which is frightening or bothersome to you?" will often encourage the patient to explore his feelings.

Patients who fear specific stimuli, including pain, tend to send this message clearly. They may say something like, "I just can't stand pain. I have low pain tolerance in my mouth."

Patients afraid of a catastrophe have fears revolving around physiological sensations, and may report fear of "choking, fainting, or having an allergic reaction."

Patients who have difficulty coping with many different kinds of events are often less able to give a specific response. They may respond with statements like, "It wasn't *that* bad, to tell you the truth, but I just couldn't make myself go again." "I don't know exactly why I hate it. I just do."

Patients who are distrustful tend to say things such as, "I'm afraid of being helpless and trapped." "I hate being made to feel guilty about my teeth." "My dentist would tell me it didn't hurt and it did!"

Frequently the issue of pain tolerance arises. Patients may mention that they have a high pain tolerance except in the mouth, or that their pain tolerance has been decreasing over the past few years. Or they may say they have low pain tolerance. Pain tolerance is the subject of much research. What is known, however, is that pain tolerance is readily modified under varying conditions. For example, in the 1950s, childbirth was considered too painful to tolerate without various nerve blocks and pain medications. Today, many women choose natural childbirth. The intervening factor? The mindset of the mother is influenced by childbirth training and practice. We will discuss in detail the importance of perception in pain tolerance in Chapter 7.

Question 4: What other kinds of things besides dentistry are you afraid of?

This question allows you to move beyond the specifics of dentistry. We find that it is important to list the most common fears—flying, heights, closed spaces, elevators, and crowds—to bring to mind other areas of concern. Your purpose is to determine the range of the patient's fears. Patients who fear specific stimuli are very rarely seriously afraid of anything besides dentistry. What do we mean by "seriously afraid?" Many of us find certain situations uncomfortable. Fears which we would categorize as serious are those which are strong enough to limit a person's activities in some way. If the patient can think of no other situation that he particularly fears, it is a reliable sign that his fears are dental-specific. Such people are among the easiest of all patients to treat once you can pinpoint the specific cause of the fears.

However, you will find that many patients are fearful of numerous situations and events. People with multiple fears generally fall primarily within the Generalized Anxiety or Catastrophe categories. You can differentiate these groups by understanding what the patient is afraid of across situations. People afraid of catastrophe will mention a fear of having the same "involuntary" physiological response that they have experienced in other situations. People with general anxiety will focus on their inability to *cope* with (mentally and emotionally tolerate) difficult stressful situations.

When a patient "admits" to other fears, it is important to explore how they affect him and; how he copes with them. You might ask an exploratory question such as: "When you find yourself in a stressful situation, how do you deal with it?" Generally anxious people respond by saying things like, "I try to ignore it," "stick my head in the sand," "avoid it." "procrastinate." The theme of their responses is that they do not cope very well. Occasionally, you will find a patient who has overcome a fear, such as of flying, of heights, or of dogs. This provides an opportunity for you to inquire about how he got over the fear. Besides being able to reinforce the idea that she can overcome her dental fear as well, you may gain some concrete ideas about how to approach the problem of their dental fear. Finally, many patients have participated in any number of "difficult or challenging" experiences such as natural childbirth, Toastmasters, self-defense courses, or mountain climbing. These require "coping skills" that can be brought to bear upon their fears of dentistry.

When a patient reports specific fears in addition to dentistry, it indicates that there is a more complex situation. A general rule is that the more situations in which the patient has difficulty coping, the more difficult it will be for you to help him learn how to tolerate dental treatment. When multiple fears are identified it is important to explore underlying commonalties. The most common theme is a fear of loss of control and a feeling of helplessness. When asked what it is they find so difficult about those situations, patients may say things like, "I guess I hate the feeling of being trapped," or "When problems start getting too big, I just get overwhelmed." Because of the central importance of the control issue we will discuss it later in this chapter when we look at paper and pencil assessment tools.

Question 6: What kinds of things could be done to make receiving care easier?

Patients who fear specific stimuli will state, "Don't hurt me!" Distrustful patients, *if* they trust you enough to respond, will talk about what they did not like about previous dental personnel and what they want you to do differently. Often their ideas are realistic or attainable. Typical responses include: "Take time to explain," "Tell me the truth," "Give me alternatives to choose from," "Let me rest," "Treat me like a person." People afraid of a medical emergency will ask you in some way to prevent their catastrophe by some technical solution such as using a different drug or different procedure. Patients with generalized anxieties will have little to recommend. They may say. "I don't know," or "Is there some drug you could use to knock me out so I don't have to know what you do?"

Question 7: How do you feel about medical care? Blood draws? Shots?

By comparing how the patient feels about medical vs. dental care you learn much about how generalized her fears are. Consider the patient who avoids physicians because they too might "want to give me a shot," or "might find something bad," in comparison with one who believes that medical injections are "no big deal." In the second situation a patient can be assured that it will be a quick and straightforward process to overcome the patient's concerns. The first patient may prove much more difficult to work with as it appears that his fears are more widespread.

Question 8: How do you feel the night/morning before you are scheduled to come in for an appointment?

Question 9: How are you likely to delay making an appointment because of your feelings about dentistry? Or to cancel it after it is made?

The two questions above help you explore what the patient was thinking before the appointment. They can elicit valuable clues about how the patient psyches himself up for a bad experience in your office. It is typical of many people with generalized anxiety to report that they don't sleep, get nervous or restless, and have other physical symptoms before an appointment. They anticipate and worry about what *might* happen. Because this patient finds it easy to avoid dental care, it is important to find out if she delays making appointments but is good about showing up, or if she is likely to fail to appear or cancel once she has made an appointment. People know what their patterns are and will tell you if asked. Obviously, a person who cancels must be treated differently from the simple avoider, for whom the principal management technique is making sure that he does not walk out of the office without another appointment. Other patients, especially those who fear specific stimuli or are distrustful, are more likely to report that "I don't worry about the dental appointment until just before I get here."

Question 10: How do you feel about the idea of taking a drug to reduce your anxiety?

Some anxious patients are very receptive to the idea. They may see a drug as "the answer" and mistakenly believe the drug will cope for them. Others are more realistic and understand that a drug is merely an aid to coping. Patients who trust you and dental care in general, but doubt their *own* abilities, are often good candidates for using anti-anxiety medications. On the other hand, if the patient is somewhat distrustful, or is fearful that dental treatment could be dangerous, or if he or she is philosophically opposed to drugs, he is unlikely to find such medications helpful.

Question 11: How do you feel about the appearance of your teeth? Explain.

Question 12: In the last two years, has the condition of your teeth caused you to cancel social activities or miss work? If yes, how much?

Question 13: Have you ever seriously considered having all your teeth pulled and getting dentures? Explain.

Question 14: Are your friends or family aware of your fears? If so, what kinds of things have they said?

The final area to be explored in the interview is what the patient perceives as the cost of illness. The questions are designed to help you gain a better understanding of the patient's dental I.Q. and the importance that he places on his teeth. Some patients state that they have thought about having their teeth pulled because they see this as the only option they could tolerate, while others actually believe that it is a good idea. Still others are terrified that their teeth will *have* to be pulled. Esthetics, of course, are very personal and a major factor in the kind of recommendations we make. The "social cost" of fear to the patient is a factor that may frequently motivate him. Patients may tolerate loss of function and inevitable changes in diet. Many patients, however, are acutely aware of their "bad smiles" and feel self-conscious to the point of limiting social contact, especially with new people. Lowering of self-esteem is not infrequent. Self-consciousness, bad breath, and the inability to smile are often seen as barriers to successful careers and relationships. These kinds of concerns do not appear to be related to any particular type of dental fear. The information obtained, however, does allow you to gain an understanding of what is important to the patient. For example, we may begin working on the anterior teeth, rather than other "more urgent" problems in order to give the patient a "high reward" during those first "high fear" appointments. The importance of modifying the treatment plan to suit the individual will be discussed in more detail later in this chapter.

Concluding the Interview

The clinician's role up to this point has been to listen in order to gain an understanding of the patient's perspective. As the interview nears a conclusion, it becomes important to tie things together and explain in general terms how you work with fearful patients. It is helpful to summarize the conceptual framework you presented before the interview. For example, "I work with a patient in two ways. First, I attempt to figure out what *I* can do to make it easier for you to accept treatment. Scheduling easier treatment first, using signal mechanisms, having rest periods, giving lots of explanations, etc., are examples of what I can do. Second, I try to ascertain what it is *you* can do for yourself to make it easier for you to get through the appointment. That is, how can I help strengthen your abilities to cope with treatment?"

It is also critical to set realistic expectations and to define what we mean by success. For example, we might say something like this: "The goal is *not* to have you feel no fear; that is, we do not expect you to become fearless. A certain degree of wariness or alertness is adaptive and normal. It is natural to be a little apprehensive when you take off in a plane. Our goal is simply to reduce your fear to a more tolerable level so you do not experience dental treatment as an emotional or mental trauma. If we can accomplish that goal I know you will be able to keep coming and seek care on a regular basis in the future. We feel this is a far more attainable goal." If you do *not* set realistic expectations about what can be accomplished, many patients will tend to feel like failures because they remain somewhat fearful despite your and their best efforts. Finally, we explain the mechanics of how the practice operates, and present the diagnostic paper and pencil measures, which are our next topic of discussion.

II. PAPER AND PENCIL ASSESSMENT TOOLS

After the interview at the Dental Fears Research Clinic, patients are asked to complete a series of questionnaires designed to obtain specific information regarding their perceptions. We administer these following the initial interview rather than before it, because we feel that if we have made the patient comfortable, we are more likely to get honest responses to questions about topics that are often perceived as embarrassing. The information that can be obtained from paper and pencil measures may also be acquired in a skillfully conducted interview. Why then use these measures? Partly because it is more efficient; but, more importantly, the responses provide a basis of comparison between patients, allowing you to assess the degree or severity of the patients' worries and fears. As Schuurs (1993) notes, every survey has limitations. However, questionnaires can serve as useful tools in the clinical setting to help you plan a management strategy. They can also be given later to determine patient progress in overcoming fear. Some of the surveys we use regularly follow.

The Dental Fear Survey

The Dental Fear Survey (DFS) has been the subject of considerable research. It has been used to provide many of the data on the prevalence of dental fear and on the specific aspects of dentistry that most people fear. The DFS is shown in Figure 4-3.

As you can see, the DFS surveys three areas pertaining to dental fear. The first two questions assess patients' reported avoidance of dentistry because of fear. Recall from Chapter 1 that 44 percent of a large sample reported having put off making an appointment because of fear and 14 percent reported having canceled one because of fear. Responses to these questions should provide you with some good indication of the patient's fear and avoidance behavior.

A second area of the DFS (questions 3 to 7) allows patients to report the degree of arousal they feel while undergoing dental treatment. As noted previously, people afraid of catastrophe are particularly attuned to their physiological states and will tend to mark the high end of these reaction scales. Consequently, this section can be particularly diagnostic for such patients. On the other hand, as we mentioned previously, self report is not always accurate. Some patients may show such arousal physically but not be aware of it themselves. For example, we recently saw a patient, diagnosed as fearful of catastrophe, whose heart rate increased from 80 to 120 beats per minute when we simply mentioned that we were going to give an injection. Even with this 50 percent increase the patient was unaware of the change. It was only after her heart rate reached 140 BPM that she reported feeling anxious! Patients who fear specific stimuli or who are distrustful may or may not report undue physiological responding.

Patient Name

Date

The first items in this questionnaire refer to various situations, feelings, and reactions related to dental work. Please rate your feeling or reaction on these items by *circling the number* (1, 2, 3, 4, or 5) of the category which most closely corresponds to your reaction.

1. Has fear of dental work ever caused you to put off making an appointment?

1	2	3	4	5
never	once or twice	a few times	often	nearly everytime

2. Has fear of dental work ever caused you to cancel or not to appear for an appointment?

1	2	3	4	5
never	once or twice	a few times	often	nearly everytime

When having dental work done:

3. My muscles become tense . . .

1	2	3	4	5
never	once or twice	a few times	often	very much

4. My breathing rate increases . . .

1	2	3	4	5
never	once or twice	a few times	often	very much

5. I perspire . . .

1	2	3	4	5
never	once or twice	a few times	often	very much

6. I feel nauseated and sick to my stomach . . .

1	2	3	4	5
never	once or twice	a few times	often	very much

7. My heart beats faster . . .

1	2	3	4	5
never	once or twice	a few times	often	very much

Following is a list of things and situations that many people mention as being somewhat anxiety or fear producing. Please rate how much fear, anxiety, or unpleasantness each of them causes you. Use the numbers 1–5, from the following scale. Make a check in the appropriate space. (If it helps, try to imagine yourself in each of these situations and describe what your common reaction is.)

1	2	3	4	5
never	once or twice	a few times	often	very much

	1	2	3	4	5
8. Making an appointment for dentistry....					
9. Approaching the dentist's office					
10. Sitting in the waiting room					

	1	2	3	4	5
11. Being seated in the dental chair.............					
12. The smell of the dentist's office.............					
13. Seeing the dentist walk in........................					
14. Seeing the anesthetic needle					
15. Feeling the needle injected......................					
16. Seeing the drill.................................					
17. Hearing the drill					
18. Feeling the vibrations of the drill............					
19. Having your teeth cleaned......................					
20. All things considered, how fearful are you of having dental work done?............					

FIGURE 4-3. Dental Fear Survey

The third section of the DFS (questions 8 to 19) allows patients to indicate how much fear each of several dental situations and procedures causes for them. This information of course is useful for the clinician to know before starting dental treatment and can provide a rational starting point for treating the dental fear.

The final question (20), a general summary, allows the patient to indicate, overall, how much fear she experiences from dentistry. Responses to this question can serve as a good overall indicator of the general state of her fear. In our research and clinical experience using this survey, we have found that most patients, whether fearful or not, report feeling relieved at being able to express their feelings concerning dentistry in this way. Many have stated that being given the opportunity to do so indicates to them that their dentist is interested in their personal well-being. Further, these responses provide a specific means by which dentists can begin or continue to discuss a patient's feelings.

Dental Beliefs Survey

Most investigations into dental fear have focused on the technical procedures that patients fear most. However, as noted earlier, this presents only a partial picture of the concerns that are involved in a patient's fears. Little attention has been directed toward the patient's subjective perceptions regarding the dentist's behavior and the process of how the care is delivered. It was for this reason that the Dental Beliefs Survey (DBS) shown in Figure 4-4 was developed (Smith *et al.*, 1984).

It is important to remember that the primary goal of the interview and the paper and pencil measures is to gain an understanding of the *patient's* perceptions about the causes of their fear. Thus the purpose of the DBS is to identify to what degree the patient perceives the *interpersonal* relationship with the dental professional as being, or contributing to, the problem. Consequently, the information obtained is both diagnostic and prescriptive. The questions are designed to help you confirm your initial diagnostic impressions as well as suggest how you, as the health care provider, can tailor your approach to best address the specific concerns of the patient.

The survey questions patients about issues that are of primary concern to patients with general anxiety or who are distrustful. Because this survey was designed to complement the Dental Fear Survey, items pertaining to patients' physiological responses and specific stimuli were not included. There are three major areas of concern explored by this questionnaire: Professionalism or Ethics (questions 1–11), Communication (questions 12–20), and Lack of Control (questions 21–28).

GETZ DENTAL BELIEFS SURVEY

The items in this questionnaire refer to various situations, feelings, and reactions related to dental work. Please rate your feelings or beliefs on these items by *circling the number* (1, 2, 3. 4, or 5) of the category which most closely corresponds to your feelings about *dentistry in general.*

	never	once or twice	a few times	often	nearly always
1. I am concerned that dentists recommend work that is not really needed.	1	2	3	4	5
2. I believe dentists say/do things to withhold information from me.	1	2	3	4	5
3. I worry if the dentist is technically competent and is doing quality work.	1	2	3	4	5
4. I have had dentists say one thing and do another.	1	2	3	4	5
5. I am concerned that dentists provide all the information I need to make good decisions.	1	2	3	4	5
6. Dentists don't seem to care that patients sometimes need a rest.	1	2	3	4	5
7. I've had dentists seem reluctant to correct work unsatisfactory to me.	1	2	3	4	5
8. When a dentist seems in a hurry I worry that I'm not getting good care.	1	2	3	4	5
9. I am concerned that the dentist is not really looking out for my best interests.	1	2	3	4	5
10. Dentists focus too much on getting the job done and not enough on the patient's comfort.	1	2	3	4	5

	never	once or twice	a few times	often	nearly always
11. I'm concerned that dentists might not be skilled enough to deal with my fears or dental problems.	1	2	3	4	5
12. I feel dentists do not provide clear explanations.	1	2	3	4	5
13. I am concerned that dentists do not like to take the time to really talk to patients.	1	2	3	4	5
14. I feel uncomfortable asking questions.	1	2	3	4	5
15. Dental professionals say things to make me feel guilty about the way I care for my teeth.	1	2	3	4	5
15. I am concerned that dentists will not take my worries (fears) about dentistry seriously.	1	2	3	4	5
17. I am concerned that dentists will put me down (make light of my fears).	1	2	3	4	5
18. I am concerned that dentists do not like it when a patient makes a request.	1	2	3	4	5
19. I am concerned that dental personnel will embarrass me over the condition of my teeth.	1	2	3	4	5
20. I believe that dentists don't have enough empathy for what it is really like to be a patient.	1	2	3	4	5

	never	once or twice	a few times	often	nearly always
21. When I am in the chair I don't feel like I can stop the appointment for a rest if I feel the need.	1	2	3	4	5
22. Dentists don't seem to notice that patients sometimes need a rest.	1	2	3	4	5
23. Once I am in the chair I feel helpless (that things are out of my control).	1	2	3	4	5
24. If I were to indicate that it hurts, I think that the dentist would be reluctant to stop and try to correct the problem.	1	2	3	4	5
25. I have had dentists not believe me when I said I felt pain.	1	2	3	4	5
26. Dentists often seem in a hurry, so I feel rushed.	1	2	3	4	5
27. I am concerned that the dentist will do what he wants and not really listen to me while I'm in the chair.	1	2	3	4	5
28. Being overwhelmed by the amount of work needed (all the bad news) could be enough to keep me from beginning or completing treatment.	1	2	3	4	5

FIGURE 4-4. *Getz Dental Beliefs Survey*

Professionalism

It is unfortunate, but true, that some fearful patients have no more trust of dental professionals than many of us have of used car salesmen. That is, we are not convinced that the other person has *our* best interests in mind. (Questions 1–11 explore these concerns) If the patient has this attitude, you need to be aware of it. It does not mean that you can not have a successful relationship with the patient. It does mean that the issue should be addressed directly. For example, well written, detailed treatment plans are usually appreciated by such patients. Additional strategies are discussed in Chapter 5 in which trust and control are discussed in greater depth.

You will note that only questions 3 and 11 relate to the patient's beliefs concerning the dentist's technical skills. Contrary to our initial expectations, we found that only a small minority of patients worry about the dentist's technical competence. Although they may be terrified of dentistry, they seldom are very concerned about the dentist "bungling it." The exceptions are generally patients who have experienced traumatic medical or dental incidents caused by an obvious operator error.

Communication

Extensive research in medicine has shown that a patient's perceived ease of communication with providers is a critical variable in determining compliance with health care recommendations and satisfaction with services (Sackett & Haynes, 1976). We believe that communication is also a crucial variable in determining the degree to which a patient's fears are decreased or exacerbated. Scott *et al.* (1984) noted, for example, that highly anxious patients were reluctant to talk with the dentist.

Questions 12 - 20 were included in the DBS to explore how well the patient believes the dentist communicates and how comfortable the patient feels in attempting to talk with the dentist. Patients might feel uncomfortable for many reasons. For some, it may be that their childhood dentist was gruff and uncommunicative. For others, it may be that the patient is not very assertive and has difficulty talking with people he perceives as authority figures. Whatever the origins of the discomfort, it is you who must make the initial outreach to these patients. It is important with the non-communicative patient to repeatedly make statements such as, "If I say anything you do not understand, let me know" or "It's important for me to know how you are feeling," or "Give me some feedback on how you feel things are going." Also bear in mind that *how* you make these comments is as important as *what* you actually say.

Hall and Edmondson (1983) note that "one of the commonest causes of dental fear has been shown to be anxiety lest the dentist should adopt a negative attitude." More than 61 percent of our new patients report that previous dentists have belittled or discounted their fears. And almost 71 percent of our patients feel that dental professionals are judgmental or make them feel guilty about their oral health.

Perhaps you feel that these reports are exaggerated. They may be. And yet they are also very understandable. As a health professional, you know that there is little to fear objectively. The procedures performed are seldom dangerous and in most cases are minimally painful. Thus, we often attempt to reassure the patient that "everything will be fine" or "it isn't that bad." Unfortunately, reassurance seldom works and patients often see it as a put-down. Similarly, because most health professionals *do* care about good health and their patients, it is easy to feel frustrated when patients act fearful, do not do what they are supposed to do, or neglect their health care. Consequently, difficulties can easily arise with a patient who is highly sensitized and frightened and who is ready to pick up on any indication of dentist frustration or disapproval. These tendencies are particularly strong in distrustful people.

Lack of Control

As noted earlier, loss of control is one of the major underlying themes in dental fear. Approximately 86 percent of the patients we see indicate that this is a critical issue for them. The following statements typify such patients' reports, "The dentist will do whatever he wants to, once he gets you in the chair." "I hate it when they hover over you. They might as well be strapping you down. I feel pinned down." "I feel at their mercy." "They always take my glasses away so I can't tell what they are doing."

Being the expert on the technical aspects of dental treatment, you do not consult the patient on how to perform a MOD on # 30. Consequently, it is very easy to ignore working with the patient to encourage his participation in treatment, which in turn might give him the perception of having no control or power. Questions 21-27 examine patients' beliefs about their ability to control what goes on during a typical treatment. At first glance, it may be difficult to believe that a patient does not feel that she could stop an appointment if she were in severe pain. And yet, this fear is frequently identified by our patients as their primary concern.

As you might guess, many patients lack self-assertiveness skills. If you question them, you will learn that they have difficulty making requests for fear of disapproval by the dentist or the hygienist. They are likely to "sit there and take it," vowing not to return because "I can't stand the thought of going back."

Question 28 focuses on a specific aspect of communication that has proven to be important in working with patients in our clinic. Gale (1972) found in his survey that the third most prevalent concern of fearful patients was the fear of "hearing bad news." Our data confirm this as one of the patient's chief concerns. This points out how extremely carefully you must communicate information, both after the initial examination as discussed in Chapter 3 and when you present the treatment plan.

Dental Cognitions Checklist

Clinicians and researchers have recently increased their attention to the thoughts or cognitions of fearful patients in an attempt to better understand how patients acquire and maintain their fears. De Jongh, *et al.* (1994) have developed a questionnaire to examine patients' anxiety expectations. As one would expect, dentally high-anxiety patients experienced significantly more negative thoughts than did low-anxiety patients. Our group is also examining patient cognitions with a newly developed checklist. It contains forty "thoughts"; the patient is asked to indicate how well each applies to her. You will note (Figure 4-5) that many of them may appear to be dramatic or exaggerated. However, it is important to remember that just this kind of thinking and feeling which maintains a phobia.

DENTAL COGNITIONS CHECKLIST _____

Name

Each item below describes a thought that some patients think to themselves about dental care. Please read each statement and indicate the degree to which it applies to you now. *I think that . . .*

Choose the answer closest to true where statement is not fully applicable.	Don't know	Not at all	Rarely	Some-times	Often	Ex-tremely
1. The needle seems so long! Like it could stick into my eye, nose, or brain.						
2. The needle might hit a nerve or something and damage it.						
3. Nothing is as painful as a needle in my mouth.						
4. The needle might break off.						
5. Medical needles are much smaller and less painful.						
6. I'm very hard to get numb.						
7. If my throat gets numb from a shot I won't be able to breathe or swallow.						
8. If I'm leaned back too far in the dental chair I get claustrophobic.						
9. When I'm in the dental chair I can't stop for a rest.						
10. Being in the dental chair can bring back bad memories from other events in my life.						
11. I can't breathe with a rubber dam.						

	Don't know	Not at all	Rarely	Some-times	Often	Ex-tremely
12. I can't swallow with a rubber dam.						
13. I might get too much radiation from the X-rays.						
14. The mercury or other metals (or plastics) might be dangerous to my health						
15. Too much topical anesthetic might make it so I could not breathe or swallow.						
16. I'm always waiting for the drill to hurt me.						
17. I'm fearful that the dentist might slip and injure me.						
18. I can't stand the sound of the drill.						
19. I can't stand the sound of having my teeth cleaned (scraped).						
20. I can't stand that burning smell when they drill on teeth.						
21. I'm allergic to some-thing—like Novocain, and it might harm me.						
22. Impressions (molds and models) make me feel like I can't swallow or breathe.						
23. Impressions (molds and models) make me feel like I will gag.						
24. X-rays make me gag.						
25. X-rays hurt.						

	Don't know	Not at all	Rarely	Some-times	Often	Ex-tremely
26. I will have losts of pain after treatment.						
27. They will find something terrible and wrong with me.						
28. I might be so scared I will do something embarrass-ing.						
29. It is so embarassing to be fearful, I might not go ahead with treatment.						
30. I get anxious before a dental appointment.						
31. I am emotionally exhausted after an appointment.						
32. I am physically exhausted after an appointment.						
33. I can't stand the sight or taste of blood.						
34. They might drill too deep.						
35. The dentist is going to say I need a root canal.						
36. I'll lose all my teeth.						
37. The numbness will not go away.						
38. The dentist will think I'm foolish or childish.						
39. I feel so guilty about letting things go, I don't deserve treatment.						
40. I'm so fearful that I'm too much trouble to treat.						

Did we miss any? Please write down any anxiety provoking or disturbing thoughts you might have relating to dental care

	Don't know	Not at all	Rarely	Some-times	Often	Ex-tremely
41.						
42.						

FIGURE 4-5. *Dental Cognition Checklist*

While the questionnaire is only in the development stage and our results are preliminary, they are quite interesting. We have, for example, been surprised by how many fearful patients with overall good dentition have expressed an extreme fear of losing all their teeth (question #36). Similarly, a high percentage of respondents have indicated that the dental environment triggers negative memories from the patient's past (question #10). At this point we recommend that you use this questionnaire only with patients who are frankly fearful and who you intend to treat.

Using Existing Records To Assess Fearful Patients

We have saved this section for last because it is the most indirect method for ascertaining if a patient is fearful. In addition, its usefulness depends, to a large degree, the quality of the charting system. A chart without notations regarding patient behavior or an accurate record of cancellations will obviously be of less use than those with more complete notes.

Over a period of time, every practice accumulates a number of patients who are "goers but haters," people who fail to respond to recall notices or are "irregular appointment makers," or patients who too frequently cancel or fail to show up for an appointment. There are of course many different reasons for patients presenting behavior problems. However, anxiety and fear about dentistry are frequently major inhibiting factors, and some patients are reluctant to openly express their fear to the dentist or auxiliaries.

The record of appointments made and kept or missed can alert the dentist to possible problems of fear. Bernstein, Kleinknecht, and Alexander (1979) reported that patients previously identified as fearful through a questionnaire mailed to them were six times more

likely to cancel or not appear for a given appointment than were
people who reported not being fearful. Records of frequent appointment changes or a sporadic, irregular distribution with two or more
years between appointments can serve as an initial sign of fearfulness, but, of course, must be supported by additional information.

Another indicator of possible fearfulness, obtainable from
records, is the patient's having had a long history of chronic illness.
In many cases, lengthy histories of illness and possibly painful and
traumatic treatment can leave one sensitized to all medical settings.
This is particularly true for children. The similarity of the dental
office and routine to other treatment environments might seem to be
one more situation in which the patient will receive painful injections or other traumatic treatments. On the other hand, some
chronically ill patients, as a result of their many medical experiences,
find their anxieties about dental treatment decrease.

A third source of information from records are clinical notes
about a patient's behavior in previous appointments. Of course,
these are valuable only if the dentist or an assistant takes the time to
record his or her impressions following an appointment. Such notation is particularly important when we consider that many patients
come for treatment or examinations sporadically. We cannot expect
to remember each patient, especially those who have not been in for
several years. Further, behavioral impressions, regularly noted, can
provide evidence of patient change over time.

Information gathered from patient records can serve as the basis
for your developing a hypothesis about the patient's level of fearfulness, which you can then follow up.

The first step is to review patient files to identify "problem" patients—those who are difficult to work with in the chair, and those
patients who have failed to follow through in treatment or regular
preventive appointments. We have found that it is very effective to
have the dentist make reactivation calls. However, in most offices,
this task will be assigned to the office receptionist.

If a staff person makes the call, she should be briefed on the procedure to follow when she contacts the patient. As we will repeatedly stress, if a dentist chooses to work with the fearful patient, the
entire staff must be brought aboard. Successful treatment requires a
team approach.

When you reach a patient by phone, a conversation might go

something like this:

Staff: Mrs. Roberts, this is Ann Jones from Dr. Humphries' office. We were going through our files and realized that we haven't seen you in a year and a half. Dr. Humphries asked me to call you about making an appointment.

Patient: Well, I had been thinking about it. I just hadn't gotten around to it. I'm a little short of cash right now. I've been real busy ... etc.

Staff: Well, I can certainly understand how that could get in the way. Dentistry is certainly an easy thing to delay. I find some people would rather do almost anything to avoid going to the dentist. Are you a person who has to force herself to go?

Patient: Yeah, I really don't like it much.

Staff: Because it is uncomfortable or scary?

Patient: Oh I know it's kind of crazy but I always get nervous thinking about it.

Staff: Oh, in that case I am glad I called. Dr. Humphries is very concerned about his patients, especially those who are nervous about going to the dentist. If you would like to make an appointment, I will make a note for Dr. Humphries to meet with you in his office to discuss with you what he can do to make it as easy as possible for you to receive care. May we set up an appointment?

With some simple telephone techniques, you are more than simply reactivating patients. You are communicating a clear message to your patients that you are concerned about their health, listening to them, and providing service.

TREATMENT PLANNING

Factors in Prioritizing Dental Treatment

How do you decide where to begin? Should you, for example,

always start with getting the patient cleaned up, moving next to the most serious dental problems, and leaving the cosmetic work until the end? Which should come first, periodontal treatment or restorative treatment? Our experience has led us to conclude that treatment planning for the fearful patient must be flexible. The order should be determined by what the patient fears and what he considers important.

The general principle guiding treatment planning is that it takes up to eight successful visits to the dentist to replace one terrifying one. Thus, a dentist should construct a treatment plan in a way that maximizes his control over the dental treatment experience in order to ensure that it is successful. For fearful patients, success is defined as the patient saying, afterwards, that the visit was not as tough as she thought it would be, and that she can come back again. Success is *not defined by whether or not a particular dental procedure is accomplished*. That is short-term thinking: such a dentist-driven definition is irrelevant to the fear problem. To phrase it another way, once seated in the chair most patients will let you complete any given procedure. That is, you can almost always win "the battle," but if the patient fails to return you will lose "the war."

Treatment should always be thought of in phases. The initial phase should include treatments designed to increase the patient's ability to tolerate treatment. For example, with a patient terrified of pain, you might initially treat a gingival infection with antibiotics, chlorhexidine rinses, and repeated coronal polishing. This will establish trust and desensitize the patient to the dental environment as well as improve his gums. Before each treatment session, you should premedicate the patient with a nonsteroidal anti-inflammatory agent or acetaminophen (paracetemol) to reduce post-operative pain. Instruct the dental hygienist to use topical anesthetic and local anesthetic injections, and to take no short-cuts in pain control. A second or third phase of treatment might include other areas of dentistry. Postpone referral to a periodontist until the patient's fears have been treated and you have established rapport.

With the patient's permission, we will often wait to extract hopeless teeth until after meeting other priorities. We have found that although there may be flare-ups, patients blame the pain on the tooth, not on the dentist, as long as he acts promptly when this occurs. Extractions are not positive steps because they do not create better looking teeth and they are considered painful by many patients. Consider putting them lower on the list of priorities with the patient's permission.

Another patient of ours was embarrassed by what she perceived as "horrible looking front teeth." In this case we began by restoring the anteriors with composite. The patient had been putting tooth-colored wax in open lesions. The procedures were simple and results good. For still another patient recently, we began treatment with chlorhexidine rinses, a simple prophylaxis and orthodontic realignment of upper anterior teeth with a fixed orthodontic appliance. We felt we could not place attractive composites until we did this. The result was a very grateful patient who had never before considered that his teeth could look so nice. Figure 4-6 shows a typical treatment plan. Note that discussion about some treatment options are postponed until phase 3.

Treatment Plan: *Jane M.*

Phase 1   Needle desensitization (1–2 hrs.)
Oral Hygiene Instruction
Fluoride, home use
Prophylaxis, 2 visits
Composites #7M, #9M
Amalgam repair #15
Re-evaluation

Phase 2   Amalgam #19 MOD
Endo #4
#4 temporary crown and post
Oral Hygiene Instruction as needed
#4 cast post and core
#4 crown

Phase 3   Recall exam and consult. Set recall interval. Discuss tx. options
#18 crown replacement?
Replace missing tooth #13. Maryland or conventional bridge? Single tooth implant?

FIGURE 4-6. Sample Treatment Plan

Presenting a Phased Treatment Plan

Dentist: As you can see, I have proposed a treatment plan involving phases of treatment. It is a go-slow approach that allows us to work together to overcome your fears and postpones some decisions until you have a better idea of what treatment here is like. What do you think?

Patient: I just want to get this over with. Can't we just schedule one or two really long appointment?

Dentist: I understand how you feel. It was a big decision to come in for treatment, and now it seems I'm dragging it out. If I were to begin with treatment of your molars now we might be able to fix one or two teeth, but the chances are very high that it would be very difficult or unpleasant for you, and you would never come back. Postponing work on those broken back teeth involves some risk that they will start hurting you. I want you to know that you can call me anytime if it bothers you, even in the evening or weekends. We will use pain medication or antibiotics to calm them down. My goal is to make this work for the long run, and find a way to make treatment more tolerable for you.

Many patients overestimate their coping skills and try to rush through the initial phase of treatment. For example, a recent patient of ours was very glib and said he was ready for an injection without a rehearsal. In the dental chair, he was fairly calm but his heart rate was over 90 beats per minute. When we coached him to breathe more slowly and to relax his muscles, his heart rate came down into the low 70's. We were able to proceed with a rehearsal and then an actual injection, which he reported as the "easiest ever." He had been aware that he was tense but unaware that his physiology was so upset.

The guiding principle for dental personnel is never to proceed with treatment when the patient is demonstrating any more than a very moderate fear response. Treatment plans need to consider the patient's level of coping. Feedback about heart rate or muscle tension often will convince a reluctant patient to go more slowly. In the case where treatment is delegated to a paraprofessional, the dentist must provide clear instruction about the treatment plan.

Often dental auxiliaries, especially dental hygienists, feel pressured to accomplish a procedure because they are afraid the patient will be reluctant to pay for an additional visit.

Postponing Decisions

Often fearful patients who have avoided the dentist need extensive treatment. In every case we divide the treatment plan into phases and present only the first phase in detail. We provide a more general picture of the later phases and indicate that decisions about some things need to be postponed until after we evaluate the success of initial treatment for fear and dental problems. This keeps us from overwhelming patients: most will make better, more dentally positive, decisions after having some success. Otherwise, such patients may choose only what they perceive as the most simple or quick procedure.

> Dentist: As a result of our discussion, I have written a treatment plan for you to read and sign acknowledging your consent to this initial phase of treatment. I have also outlined in global terms the type of treatment that will be involved in the later phases. Do you have any questions?
>
> Patient: Don't I need a bridge to replace my missing back teeth?
>
> Dentist: I am not sure what to recommend right now. In the first phase of treatment we will try to stabilize your periodontal status and once I see the results of that treatment we will meet again and I will propose options about your missing teeth. Right now I do not feel I have enough information to make a thoughtful recommendation.

Avoid getting dragged into discussions of procedures that will occur far in the future. If the first phase of treatment involves initial periodontal therapy, describe that. If in the midst of that explanation, the patient asks about root canal therapy, gently suggest that you will explain that when the time comes to make a decision, not now. Fearful patients often jump around in such a conversation and your job is to keep it on track.

A written plan for Phase 1 treatment, including the prices, is always a good idea. In addition, a general written description of the longer-term goals can be included. On the other hand, avoid long lists of treatments that encompass multiple phases. These will overwhelm many patients and may create a barrier to starting treatment. In addition, in many cases it is simply unrealistic to expect to get true "informed consent" from a patient with an extensive treatment plan when it is presented all at once. Most patients will also appreciate your help in predetermining their insurance benefits and estimating their copayment. Very often our longer-term avoiders of care have no idea how dental prepayment systems work.

There are often two parts to the message that dental personnel send in presenting treatment options. The first part emphasizes the benefits of treatment. "Your teeth will look better." "You'll be able to save your teeth." The second part involves lowering barriers to treatment. "We will go slowly and let you have plenty of rest breaks." "I will teach you how to relax your muscles while you are in the dental chair." "I have a portable CD player you can listen to while I am working." Our experience is that the second part, lowering the barriers to treatment, is the key to success in working with the new patient. Recall the approach-avoidance gradiants discussed in Chapter 1. When we question our patients closely we find that they already know about the benefits of dentistry and have no doubt that they would benefit if only they believed they could tolerate treatment. Thus, a fundamental principle in presenting treatment plans is communication that lowers barriers to entering treatment.

Stressing the benefits of treatment in order to get someone to go ahead can inadvertently employ fear and guilt-raising communication. For example, "If you don't proceed with treatment now, your periodontal disease may get worse and you'll lose your teeth." It is far better to underplay this type of message as most of these patients are already worried enough. Many become paralyzed and unable to make a decision in the face of this type of pressure.

Word Pictures

There is often confusion between using metaphors and analogies to help patients better understand the arcane world of dental treatment planning and "talking down" to patients. It is our experience that patients appreciate a scientific medical explanation of their condition. It is appropriate to define caries and periodontal disease as bacterial infections. It is appropriate to differentiate between teeth with broken cusps caused by wear and tear and those with frank dental caries. At the same time, explaining that endodontic treatment is like washing out a cut reduces the scariness of the procedure while communicating a fairly accurate account of what actually happens. Similarly, you can draw an analogy between periodontal disease and diabetes, by explaining that they are both chronic, but with effort, controllable conditions. However, neither is "curable," and both require ongoing attention and maintenance.

Real Pictures

Use radiographs, models, drawings, or intra-oral videos to reinforce your presentation. We often suggest that patients bring along a spouse or "significant other" to serve as a second set of ears during this discussion. Later on, this person may help the potential patient understand the merits of your step-wise approach. We encourage the patient to take the information home and think about whether or not the approach makes sense for him. Cajoling patients into accepting treatment plans leads to passive acceptance and later failure. Many distrustful patients will become angry when approached in this manner. We encourage second opinions, especially in this type of patient. Most patients, faced with the pressure a dentist can generate, will accede to treatment only to cancel or "no show" later.

Treatment Options

One final point about treatment planning. We have observed that many dentists under-treat fearful patients because the patients are difficult to work with. Failure to address fear and anxiety issues frequently results in compromises and poor care. Our experience suggests that careful planning will result in a patient who is relatively easy to care for and is maintained in practice for many years. Assume that the patient will be around for many years and save some less immediate care (elective crowns, posterior bridges, etc.) for a follow-up period. Trying to present too many options early on may be overwhelming. Consider terminating the initial phase of treatment as follows:

Dentist: I am extremely pleased with your progress. All the broken and decayed teeth you came in with are repaired. More importantly, your gums are healthy and you have learned how to prevent further problems from occurring.

Patient: Yes, I'm really happy with how things have gone. I don't think I could have done this with any other dentist.

Dentist: Thank you. When I see you in two months for a checkup on your gums, we can talk about making you a permanent crown for your front tooth and discuss the options about replacing your missing teeth on the bottom. You can think about it in the meantime.

Postponing decisions, and short initial recalls help the patient become accustomed to regular visits and is important in preventing the return of fear.

CONCLUSION

In this chapter we examined the process of how to assess a patient's concerns about receiving dental treatment and how those fears can be categorized or diagnosed.

There is no single sign of behavior that will point to a definite diagnosis. Each piece of information you collect must be placed in context with every other to gradually form a picture of the problem. That is why we emphasize that each person in the office has a role as an observer, from the time the receptionist first speaks with the patient on the telephone and on through the treatment appointments. Your task is to find the answers to two questions: First, what is the patient afraid of, and how does he respond to the fear? Second, what must I do to address those concerns so that this experience is different from his earlier ones? In answering these questions you will be able to determine if you feel comfortable treating the patient, or if you feel that he or she should be referred to a more experienced practitioner or mental health specialist. The interview questions, observation of the signs of anxiety, and the paper and pencil questionnaires are simply tools to help you answer those questions. With a working understanding of the four types of fear, you can fit the pieces of the puzzle together to reach a diagnosis and select the treatment strategies discussed later in the text that have the highest probability of success. Diagnosis is an inexact science at best. However, with practice, our accuracy improves. And what if you initially misdiagnose, or choose a strategy which seemingly does not work? The same rules and procedures apply in this area as they do in any other; you ask further questions, re-analyze the information you have already obtained, and try the next strategy.

Finally, we discussed some basic principles of treatment planning which can help phase in the proposed care in a way to increase the probability that the patient will accept and begin treatment.

QUESTIONS AND EXERCISES

1. Describe two main differences between patients fearful of catastrophe and those with generalized anxiety.

2. Have every patient scheduled for restorative work on a particular day and complete the Dental Fear Survey and Dental Beliefs Scale. How many would you predict have ever put off making an appointment due to fear? How many would you predict have ever canceled an appointment due to fear? Record the patients' responses and evaluate the differences from your predictions. If there are differences, how do you account for them?

3. What types of patients are more likely to be identified by the Dental Beliefs Survey rather than by the Dental Fears Survey? What are the differences between them?

4. After your patients have completed the Dental Fears Survey and the Dental Beliefs Scale, ask them how they felt about completing these forms. Did they find it of interest, an annoyance? Also, ask them if they think it would be a good idea to have patients routinely fill them out.

5. What are the advantages of presenting proposed treatment in phases?

6. What are some particular concerns to consider when presenting a treatment plan to a distrustful patient?

FIVE

The Foundation of Psychological Management:

Specific Strategies to Enhance Trust and Control

- Building a Trusting Relationship
- Providing Control
- Informational Control
- Behavioral Control
- Retrospective Control
- Special Concerns for Distrustful Patients

Introduction

This chapter provides one of the foundations for successful management of the patient. No matter how skilled the clinician is in behavioral or pharmacological management, the outcome will be in doubt when the patient does not trust the clinician or have the type or level of control he wants.

Patient satisfaction with dental treatment has its roots in the interpersonal skills of the dentist (Hittelman, 1983; Kress, 1988). Interpersonal communication skills as a means to alleviate patient anxiety has been a major focus of Friedman and his colleagues (1989).

Most patients trust their dentists. Dentistry is a respected profession with its own code of ethics. On the other hand, there are some who are distrustful. Who are these folks? What do we need to do to be successful with them?

Distrust occurs when we fail to establish rapport with patients, belittle their fears or self-care habits, or otherwise fail to anticipate or respond to their concerns. The distrustful patient may appear angry, want everything in writing, and wish to have a friend or spouse in the operatory. He may want a mirror so he can watch every move you make and he may request a lot of information. This patient is alert and sensitive to your personal and professional demeanor, your competence and ethics, and your assessment of him.

Distrust often originates from direct experiences: "The dentist wouldn't stop when I told him it hurt to drill," or "The dentist didn't give me the information I needed." Other common presenting complaints: "The dentist is always in a rush, he doesn't know me as a person" or "I wanted to have my teeth cleaned in two short appointments and the dentist said I was being silly."

The patient's previous experiences may also result in a perception of dentists as lacking caring or competence. Patient reports concerning ethics usually focus on issues related to over-treatment or to a narrow focus on financial issues.

On the other hand, distrust can originate indirectly: "My mother told me dentists don't really care about the people they treat, all they are interested in is money." Or distrust may stem in part from non-dental experiences such as unsuccessful medical procedures or poor rapport with physicians that generalizes to dentists.

While most distrust of dentists is a simple response to avoid feeling vulnerable (as they were before), it is important to note that there are psychiatric issues that relate to trust. People who have been sexually or physically abused may not readily trust dental personnel of the same sex as the abuser. Moreover, there are paranoid individuals who, usually beginning in early adulthood, interpret the actions of others as deliberately demeaning or threatening. They do not usually confide in others for fear of revealing information that will be used against them. Such people are usually argumentative, appear to be "cold," and have no sense of humor. While dentists do not usually find it difficult to establish trust with most patients, even some who are initially distrustful of dentists, it is beyond the expertise of most dental personnel to establish trust with those who are paranoid.

BUILDING A TRUSTING RELATIONSHIP

We will now discuss the key elements of building a trusting relationship. They are: building rapport, two-way communication, expressing concern, demonstrating competence and ethics, and the involvement of significant others.

Building Rapport

You must establish rapport with the apprehensive patient as early as possible. We believe that fearful patients form impressions of the dentist in the first few minutes of an initial encounter. Thus, the dentist should spend the first three to five minutes of this appointment trying to learn about the patient. A common complaint of patients referred to the Dental Fears Research Clinic at the University of Washington is that the "dentist didn't know me as a person." The dentist should devote most of this time to listening to concerns and exploring patient interests. Rapport is a harmonious relationship; the goal is to make the patient comfortable while getting acquainted. This does not legitimize "small talk" about the weather, current events, the local sports team, and so on. Instead, rapport is likely to be encouraged when you discuss the patient's concerns early on and demonstrate real interest in her life and how her situation might impact treatment. The ability to ask a question that requires more than a yes/no answer and just listen is extremely important at this time. Make notations on the patient's chart about his concerns and special interests. Refer to them each time you meet with the patient. For example, remembering that her boss is not very understanding about letting her leave work for appointments or that she has her invalid mother living at home and must plan ahead to make sure supervised care is available is very helpful in building rapport. With a distrustful patient, you must renew and reinforce rapport at each visit. It cannot be taken for granted and must be an important consideration at each appointment. Occasionally, you will need extra time beyond the initial appointment to establish and then maintain rapport.

Our experience suggests that the competent yet caring professional is best for the distrustful patient. What does this mean? First, be on time and be prepared and ready to treat this patient. One patient we recently treated complained that her previous dentist did not have her insurance predetermination in hand when he discussed her care plan. Do not interrupt the patient or take a condescending tone. Patients who feel vulnerable are often acutely sensitive to discourtesies. Do not call the patient by his or her first name until you have permission to do so. For some patients, especially those sensitive to status, it may be useful to offer the option of calling you by *your* first name.

Second, examine your environment. What is on the walls, what is your music? What does it project? Your reception area gives patients an impression of the sort of relationship they will have with you. Try to warm up the environment. Decorations and expensive artwork are not necessary. A few pictures of your family or of you holding a string of fish, or your child's artwork, can give even the most angry patient an image of the dentist as a real person. Greet the patient outside the operatory. These are important sources of non-verbal communication.

Third, remember to make eye contact and be sensitive to your posture. Demonstrate your concern by your non-verbal gestures. Touching the patient gently with permission is much better than just verbal reassurance. Do not hurry. Hurrying, which is a major patient complaint about dentistry, conveys to the patient that you are not interested in him. Lean toward the patient when you are trying to show interest in what he is saying.

With fearful patients it is very easy to forget that most patients have very positive opinions about dentists. It is important not to take personally the indication of distrust from an anxious person. Try, instead, to ask the patient how you can facilitate his care, how you can improve the experience. Establish positive expectations. Let the patient know you want to hear his thoughts, feelings, and reactions so you will be able to help him have a good experience. It is also appropriate to openly acknowledge that his past experiences have not been positive and that you want your experience with him to be different. Such a conversation might sound like this:

Patient: I'm afraid to let you look at my gums. The last dentist really made me feel guilty for letting them get this bad.

Dentist: I understand you are concerned about being put down. I want to focus on the future, not the past. After I look at your gums, I will try to give you a full explanation of the situation and recommendations you can think about. You can ask questions, then you can decide what you want to do.

A final element in building rapport is to model openness. As we have just noted, fearful patients are afraid of being put down. Positive statements by you which reveal something about yourself are useful.

Dental Assistant: You know, I used to be anxious about going to the dentist.

Patient: Really?

Dental Assistant: I have always been uptight about sitting in the chair. But I found out that our dentist really tried to get to know me and understand my fears. Now I'm really comfortable.

Such statements allow the patient to be herself and to express concerns about treatment without fear of embarrassment or belittlement. It is important to note (and easy to forget) that the behavior of the staff is very important in forging positive relationships with fearful patients. Most of the work in establishing rapport is routinely done by the staff in the office. Your staff may be very competent in this area. A little training in this area can go a long way.

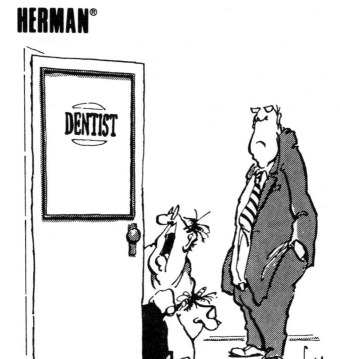

"Grab his legs!"

Two-Way Communication

Two-way communication is essential in your work with the distrustful patient. These patients need to learn that they can exercise some personal control in what they perceive as a dangerous situation. The vehicle is communication.

Not long ago this type of anxious patient would have spent a lot of time rinsing his mouth and spitting into the cuspidor. Patients will often use this type of maneuver as a substitute for telling you what the problem is. As a clinician you must tell the patient that he needs to let you know how he is doing. The distrustful patient feels that he cannot control what the dental professional will do. He feels powerless and like a victim. You might look at the solution to this as *assertiveness training* for the patient. In this setting, assertiveness is simply being able to communicate one's likes and dislikes and questions with dental personnel.

Another example of distrust occurs when the patient continually asks: "Why is this treatment going to be better?" The best response is, "Please tell me what you would like me to do to make treatment a good experience for *you*." You may also need to tell the patient which areas he should give you feedback about. These preferences are important to the success of treatment. For example, the non-assertive patient may not feel comfortable telling the dentist that the anesthesia is not completely effective, that he gets dizzy when the chair is tipped all the way back, or he does not understand the treatment plan or the costs of treatment. Unasked questions add considerably to distrust.

Imagine how you would feel as a patient if you had to sit there and bear the discomfort and couldn't say anything. Wouldn't your apprehensiveness grow? Many patients will simply fail to report being hurt out of concern that the dentist may make light of their discomfort. A previous dentist may have said "Sit still, it will only be a little bit longer," or "It's not very uncomfortable. This isn't a very bad cavity." Try to reverse roles and imagine yourself as your patient under these circumstances.

Helping patients become comfortable in communicating their desires will reduce the likelihood of uncompleted treatment plans and failed appointments, and will ultimately reduce your frustration. Perhaps some examples will be helpful.

The first patient is an older woman who has generally taken good care of her teeth but now has a failing lower fixed bridge. She is already partially edentulous in the lower arch. She visited a prosthodontist who strongly recommended reconstruction of the upper and lower teeth, including fixed and removable appliances.

She had her teeth cleaned by the dentist's hygienist and then reported to the office on three separate occasions to begin restorative treatment. *Each time she would not allow the dentist to begin.* Nevertheless, in none of the visits did she tell the dentist that she was not prepared to go ahead with this extensive treatment. It simply did not meet her needs, but she was not assertive enough in her communication with the dentist to ask questions or to tell him that she didn't want to go ahead.

We recently received a letter about another patient from a dentist who was puzzled and frustrated over losing a $6,000 case. The patient had expressed her fears initially, and the dentist recommended some specialty treatment before the crown and bridge. While the patient complied, she found the specialist impersonal and had questions about the cost. Although she returned several times for consultations and agreed to begin the crown and bridge, she changed dentists before treatment could begin. Her assessment: she felt that she had no say at all in who provided treatment and began to "feel abused."

Expressing Concern

We communicate concern in two basic ways: verbally and non-verbally. Non-verbal communication of concern, or warmth, is expressed through such behavior as head nodding, eye contact, appropriate facial expressions, and other signs of interest and attention.

Verbal expressions of concern are commonly reassurances, or the attempt to reassure someone. "Don't worry, Mrs. Jones, everything will be all right." While dental personnel who express such sentiments are trying to communicate their concern for patients, their efforts may have the *opposite* effect. Especially when reassurance is provided prematurely, as a kind of knee-jerk response to patient upset, it is often interpreted by patients as denying or ignoring their feelings.

Alternative behaviors involve responding to feelings and questioning patients about their feelings and concerns. Responding to feelings involves being a good listener and reflecting the patient's feelings. For example, if a patient said, "I'm not sure I want to go ahead with the surgery today," your feeling response would indicate to the patient that you heard his expression of concern. You might say, "You feel worried." Note that when you respond to feelings you mirror or express the same feeling as the patient.

Questioning for feeling and showing concern involve direct demonstrations of caring. "Let me know if something is bothering you" (I care). "Are you okay?" "Can I do something to make you more comfortable?" Such statements are usually appreciated and enhance trust. On the other hand, nothing can generate distrust like put-downs (e.g., "You're acting childishly.") and criticisms, no matter how well meaning or benign (e.g., "You're not taking good care of yourself."). Similarly, coercion or pressure to accept your treatment plan should be avoided, as should giving advice in general. One last note: while expressing caring through humor can be useful in lifting patients' spirits and providing distraction, it can backfire, especially with distrustful patients.

Demonstrating Competence and Ethics

Some fearful patients attribute their fears to perceptions or experiences relating to the incompetence or lack of ethics of previous dentists. For such patients it is very important for you to behave in an extremely organized and professional manner, and to make explicit the steps you take in diagnoses and treatment planning. Collect information from the patient in a deliberate, systematic manner, carefully take notes, and contact the patient's previous dentist and physician when appropriate for diagnostic and treatment planning reasons. Thank the patient for sharing information. Make it clear to the patient that you will not make off-the-cuff diagnoses or recommendations. Emphasize that you will gather all the needed information and that you need time to plan. Do not give in to patient pressure to come up with an "immediate answer" or solution to the patient's problem.

You may also enhance trust by providing detailed, written treatment plans spelling out the treatment options. It is helpful to include costs and the advantages and disadvantages of each option. Paradoxically, you often enhance trust by suggesting that the patient seek a second opinion. This shows that you are confident of the diagnosis and treatment plan and not overly eager to proceed.

Including a Significant Other

Another way to generate trust is to encourage patients to bring another person to treatment planning discussions and to dental treatment appointments. A person who is afraid of being hurt, or simply needs reassurance, may wish to bring a trusted friend or relative into the operatory. There is no reason not to allow this! In another setting Sosa and others reported in 1980 that in healthy Guatemalan women, a supportive lay woman giving birth, a "doula," had a positive effect on the length of labor, rate of perinatal problems, and mother-neonate interaction. This added social support may have a positive reassuring effect on dental patients as well.

At the University of Washington, we recently treated a young, intelligent woman who initially was angry and distrustful. She reported a series of unpleasant experiences with previous physicians and had not been to a dentist for more than ten years. She requested that a friend be present in the operatory during the examination. Our staff acknowledged her concern and gave the friend the assistant's stool at chairside. In retrospect, the friend was our biggest advocate and provided considerable encouragement. Having a "significant other" present provides both social reinforcement and another set of ears and eyes to help the patient interpret the dental experiences.

PROVIDING CONTROL

Providing the patient with some control is essential in working with patients who are afraid of dental procedures. For example, Logan and her colleagues (1991) found that when perceived control over the dentist was low and the desire for control was strong, subjects showed a marked fear response. In subsequent work, Baron, Logan, and Hoppe (1993) found that the discrepancy between felt and desired levels of control to be important for pain report during root canal therapy. Averill (1973), Thompson (1981), and Miller (1979) have defined four categories of control that may be helpful. (See Chapter 2 for discussion of these as etiologic factors in dental fear).

The first category involves giving *information*. Most fearful patients like to know what sensations will be forthcoming. For example, we tell our patients that they will feel "pressure" during injections. Moreover, it is useful to include not only what the patient can expect to happen, but also what he can do about it when it occurs: "Sometimes patients experience difficulty breathing during an impression; it's better if you concentrate on breathing through your nose..." There is vast psychological literature indicating that aversive events are much less stressful when they are predictable (Lazarus, 1966; Elliot, 1969; Seligman *et al.*, 1971). Overall, specific information and explanation are useful for fearful patients.

The second type of control involves *cognitive* change. This has to do with how patients think about the situation they are in; the "meaning" they give the event. Patients may believe that they cannot control what they think about events. In such situations, they may anticipate many negative occurrences, which become self-fulfilling prophecies. Cognitive control strategies such as distraction and guided imagery work well with these patients. These strategies will be discussed with other coping strategies in Chapter 6.

A third strategy involves enhancing *behavioral control*. Here the patient is given the opportunity to influence what is actually going on. For example, "Raise your hand when you're ready for us to start."

The last strategy is *retrospective control*. This is essentially *post-hoc* explanation. While a procedure may be aversive (e.g., tightening an orthodontic ligature), after it is over the dentist explains that the patient's pain is a protective mechanism telling the dentist not to tighten the wire any further. Such an explanation may serve to lessen anticipation of subsequent appointments.

In this chapter we discuss three types of control: informational, behavioral, and retrospective control. Informational control involves explanation, behavioral control involves primarily signal mechanisms. These control mechanisms give the fearful patient a way to cope with the stress of a dental procedure.

INFORMATIONAL CONTROL

How you prepare and deliver of information to patients who are about to undergo a stressful procedure is extremely important. Do not surprise a patient. After a patient defines a procedure as stressful, the key issues are:

1. What and how much to tell the patient
2. When to tell him
3. How to tell him

How much and what. There are three parts of this issue. *First*, information about technique. Generally, dentists tell patients too much about technical dental procedures and too little about their safety and comfort. Technique should be described concisely in lay terms. "In the root canal treatment I carefully remove decay and infection that has involved the roots of the teeth." "When I do a filling in this tooth I will mainly be removing the old silver." *Second*, safety. Immediately before the event, tell patients what to expect so they know how to cooperate, and what measures you are taking for their safety. "The rubber dam is placed so you won't swallow any of the debris or dental materials while I'm working." "Your tongue is protected with the dam in place." It is extremely useful to leave the patient's glasses on. Without the ability to see, many patients feel out-of-control and vulnerable. *Third*, suggestions for comfort. Tell patients that you do some procedures for their comfort. Tell them how to respond if they are uncomfortable. "The topical anesthetic ointment will make your gums more comfortable while I clean this area. Please tell me if you want me to use it anywhere else."

When to give information. Basic information outlining general strategies is appropriate during case presentations. But never give complex explanations, such as detailing each step of a procedure or describing the feeling of a forceps extraction, far in advance of treatment unless they are requested. Misunderstandings at that point will lead to more fearful anticipation. It is more important to provide the information just before the stressful procedure.

It is important to note that some patients prefer minimal information; providing them with detailed information will increase their upset. Do not give all patients the same information. Identify their preferences.

How you give information. When telling a patient about a dental procedure, include all the senses. It is important to describe what the procedure may smell and feel like, what the instruments may sound like, and what the patient may see reflected in the dentist's safety glasses. Be very careful about the words you use.

Take care in making requests to the chairside assistant. Patients often interpret what the dentist says literally. An "enamel hatchet" could be a large object more appropriate to the woods or battlefield than to their mouths. Euphemisms are not difficult to find. Patients who fear specific procedures often have had no recent experience with the procedure. They have avoided dentistry for so long that the "avoidance" gradient is easily lowered with a few successful experiences, allowing them to approach the feared procedure in the future. Describing your procedure as "different" from the past is useful. We often use the analogy between old propeller airplanes and commercial jets of the present, or the differences between the engines of an old '57 Chevy and a new Saturn. We stress to the patient that dental procedures are now improved, that we are concerned about their experience, and that they have new coping skills they can apply to successfully tolerate the experience. Support and encouragement, with information, work especially well if the patient has not received treatment since childhood.

Tell-Show-Do

This procedure, so successful with children, is also appropriate for adults. Such a procedure teaches patients about "new" sensations.

Dentist: The first part of the cleaning procedure involves using an instrument to feel the surfaces of your teeth. Let me *show* you what I will do on this model (demonstrate). Perhaps you could hold the mirror and watch while I feel one of your teeth just as I did on the model? Can you feel the rough spot that my instrument is touching? That's tartar, or calculus, and it is what causes tooth decay.

Patient: Yes it feels very big.

Dentist: Yes it does, it comes off easily (demonstration). When your gums heal they will be more comfortable. I will be feeling around each of the teeth very carefully to check for rough areas on your tooth. Then, I'll be cleaning them to make them smooth. When I'm doing this, it may sound a little strange and you will feel the instrument rubbing on your tooth but it will not be uncomfortable.

Another situation where *tell-show-do* works involves the high speed drill. The major problems with drilling are noise, vibration, and water. We explain the noise of the drill and water and the high speed vacuum as a cacophony. We ask patients to experience this "music" before we begin. And at this point we demonstrate the noises and everything spinning around outside of the mouth. This eliminates surprise.

While you are working, it is useful to keep the patient informed about how long the procedure will take and how far you have progressed. This kind of information keeps the patient in touch with reality and reduces her anxiety. It also helps keep you on schedule.

It's also helpful to ask several times during the appointment whether or not she would like to look at the work being done. Patient willingness to look at work in progress is a sign that fear is abating.

Another aspect of *watching in the mirror* is ability of some patients to dissociate their fear from what they are observing. From the patient's perspective, it is as if the work is being performed on another person. Emotional responses that interfere with treatment may thus be minimized. The mirror is a handy tool.

Time-structuring

Just knowing how long a procedure will last gives the patient some control; moreover, when you break up a procedure into small pieces and let the patient know how long each piece will last, you give the patient control and facilitate his coping. While many fearful patients believe they can not tolerate dental drilling or curettage, most report that they can tolerate a few seconds of aversive dental stimuli. For example, when we are about to drill on a tooth we tell the patient that we will drill for only one second—to a count of one. We remind the patient to identify a coping strategy she will use (see Chapter 6) and then ask her to signal that she is ready (see Behavioral Control). We then count "one" while the handpiece touches the tooth. If the patient finds the experience tolerable, we repeat it and lengthen the count from one to two or three. The count quickly can go from three to five or even ten. Rests between counts rarely last longer than 30 seconds. Very little time is lost when we prep teeth this way. Injections may proceed in a similar fashion. Before the procedure the dentist or hygienist will tell the patient that the procedure will take a given number of seconds and that it is possible to stop at any point should the patient signal (see Behavior Control). After inserting the needle, the dentist or hygienist tells the patient when the procedure is half and then three-quarters completed. If the patient indicates discomfort or otherwise signals, the clinician either stops pushing anesthetic or momentarily withdraws the syringe from the patient's mouth. These procedures are appropriate for both adults and children.

BEHAVIORAL CONTROL

When you introduce the importance of control to patients, you can use the analogy of removing a splinter. Most of us can use a needle to remove a splinter from our finger. While it is uncomfortable, few would describe it as unbearable or intensely painful. It is bearable because *we* control the needle and the importance attributed to it. The discomfort of a dental procedure is no worse; only the *control* aspect is different. Always frame explanations in terms that patients can understand: a religious person, a businessman, or a punk rocker would require different metaphors.

Signaling

Many patients fear not being able to control what the dentist is doing. Our view is that simply telling a patient he may signal that something hurts is not enough. For the fearful patient, active training by the dentist to instill and reinforce control is required. Signals as a control mechanism have positive implications for the success of treatment. When a patient accepts responsibility for indicating to the dentist his status, he will have overcome much of his helplessness. The patient's perception of control is critical.

Patients are not accustomed to participating in treatment. We find that encouraging them to watch procedures is helpful. It makes them more aware of what's going on and increases their control. Remember to allow patients to keep their eyeglasses on, and to use the patient mirror. Even if they decline, they know the opportunity is available.

Signal mechanisms are especially helpful to the patient with a rubber dam in place; simple hand or finger signals, a button connected to some kind of light or noisemaker, and a pad of paper and a pencil are useful. Initially the patient may interrupt often. That is a positive event. For example in this scenario:

Patient: (Raises the hand)

Dentist: Are you having some discomfort?

Patient: (writes on pad) I need to go to the bathroom.

Dentist: I'm glad you told me. We have a stopping place just ahead and then you should be able to go. Is that OK?

Patient: Yes. Thank you.

Some patients will interrupt treatment frequently during the first several visits. It is critical that you not show impatience at these interruptions. As patients become more comfortable and eager for treatment to proceed, they will interrupt less often. Realizing that "the dentist won't get mad at me" reduces the patient's feeling of anxiety and guilt.

Signaling Readiness to Proceed. Signaling is useful for stopping treatment in case of pain or need for a break, but there is an even more effective signal strategy. Using it to indicate a readiness to *proceed* is a more positive aspect of encouraging control. In this example we ask the patients to tell us when they are ready for an injection.

Dentist: I'm going to be using this fruit flavored topical ointment to make your skin numb around this tooth. (Pointing) I'm going to smear some of the ointment on the skin above the tooth, and I'd like you to let me know when you can feel the numbness or tingling or cold or warm feeling that the topical anesthetic provides. That's when we know the area is numb.

Patient: (after a minute) Yes, now I can feel the numbness.

Dentist: Good, are you ready to move on to the injection.

Patient: One more breath, and then let's do it.

Few, if any patients, will fail to respond to these suggestions. Be sure to reinforce the patient for being ready to proceed. If they do fail, it is a sign to rethink your diagnosis of the problem.

Failing to Respond to Signals. Many patients complain that the dentist does not respond to verbal or other signals. If you have instructed a patient to give a signal for needing a rest break, you must honor your commitment. Remember that with the fearful patient, control is paramount. Not living up to your end of this implied social contract reduces patient trust.

Remember, too, that relinquishing control of these aspects of treatment is technically unimportant.

Behavioral Strategies Useful with the Injection

It's ironic that the very procedure that allows patients to be treated virtually free of pain is the one that they often fear the most. Many are afraid of the pain of the injection; others exaggerate the extent of the needle penetration. We'll discuss these basic problems here. Other aspects of the use of anesthetics and reactions to anesthetics are in Chapter 8.

It often is helpful to begin exposure to anesthetic injection by using an infiltration rather than a block. We do this because the results are very predictable and the pain of injection is minimal with careful technique. However, similar procedures can be followed for injections in any area. We are not reluctant to give injections in any part of the mouth at the initial treatment visit, if that is what is needed. This includes palatal injections and others that the dentist may perceive as painful. The following scenario describes how we prepare our patients through information and behavioral control.

Patient: I'm really concerned about the injection.

Dentist: I understand your concern. The major source of discomfort with injections is the pressure. The needle puncture itself lasts only a second and generally patients don't even feel it because we use topical anesthetic on the skin. If I go very slowly, you will find that the pressure created by the anesthetic in the tissue is not painful. However, you will always feel the pressure. That's good, because

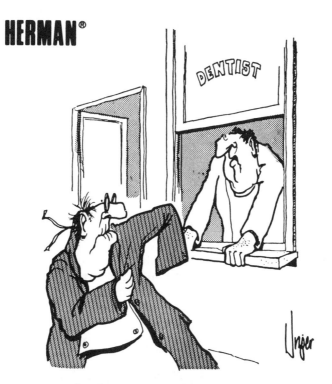

HERMAN®

"What happened! Did I touch a nerve?"

it will remind you of the anesthetic working. I'd like you to imagine, first of all, that your hand or your foot has gone to sleep. I think you can probably remember what that feels like can't you?

Patient: Yes.

Dentist: Imagine that it's gone to sleep and that it feels very heavy and numb but it doesn't hurt. Can you picture that?

Patient: Yes.

Dentist: OK, I would like to put some topical anesthetic ointment on your tongue to see if you can feel the numbness in your tongue.

Patient: (after 15 seconds) Yes, I can really feel it.

Dentist: OK, that's very good. Now I'd like to dry a spot on your gums and put on some of the topical ointment. Sometimes it's harder for patients to be able to feel it here, but I'd like you to try and see if you can feel it. Even if you can't feel it, you know that the same feeling of numbness is going to exist in the skin. I'll paint some on now and you take just a moment and tell me if and when you can feel the anesthetic.

Patient: (After 30 seconds) Yes, 1 can feel the numbness now.

Dentist: Very good. It's difficult for some patients to feel this. It's good that you're able to do it. Now, I'm going to lift your lip and administer some additional anesthetic. The skin is very numb. You will experience some pressure, which won't be painful. And as you feel that pressure, you will feel the spreading of the numbness. (Needle inserted)

Dentist: I'm going very slowly. I'm about half done now (about 30 seconds) The slower I go, the more comfortable it is for you. I'm three-quarters done. Now I'm done. You looked like you felt pretty comfortable.

Patient: Yes I didn't feel the needle at all.

Dentist: But you did feel the pressure, didn't you.

Patient: Yes, but I knew what to expect. And I can feel the numbness spreading.

Note that good technique is required. Needles should be placed carefully and the anesthetic administered slowly. Thirty seconds or more are required to empty the first 1.8-ml cartridge. Pressure anesthesia or additional topical anesthetic should always be used wherever the dentist or hygienist anticipates that there may be discomfort. Our reading of the situation is that the key variables are preparation (using the topical as above) and care in injecting slowly. In our view, other factors such as anesthetic temperature or needle gauge are relatively unimportant.

One additional word about needles. One advantage of beginning with an infiltration in the anterior is the short needle used. Usually after that first good experience with an anesthetic, we try to show the syringe to the patient. For some patients it is helpful to do this step before we give them their first injection. At this time we show them that little of the needle actually penetrates the skin and explain that the long needle is for safety. With this example patients will generalize and then anticipate, even if the injection is a mandibular block, that the needle does not penetrate very far. This will help them to be more comfortable with the injection procedure. See chapter 8 for further discussion on needle phobia.

Dentist-planned Rest Breaks

Dentist-planned breaks are extremely important, especially for the patient who is unassertive or the patient who has an unrealistic expectation of his ability to tolerate dental procedures, These short respites are important to ensure that minor discomfort does not become unbearable. The following is an example of the use of planned rest breaks:

> The patient, a woman in her late forties, had much previous treatment. She suffers from chronic back pain and has difficulty sitting in the chair comfortably for long periods. Her previous treatment experiences were traumatic, and she sought care from the Dental Fears Research Clinic after avoiding treatment for a defective bridge, several failed endodontic treatments, and at least one symptomatic, previously untreated tooth.
>
> Because of scheduling we could not treat the patient in a timely way, so a referral was made. With the patient's con-

sent, we arranged for the endodontist to see her that day. We gave him explicit instructions to structure the appointments with 5-minute periods of treatment followed by one-minute rest breaks out of the chair, and to give the patient control over the length of the rest breaks. With this simple strategy, the patient received care in a humane manner and gave us glowing reports of her treatment.

RETROSPECTIVE CONTROL OR DEBRIEFING

As noted previously, retrospective control involves discussion of what already has happened. Even though these discussions occur *post-hoc* they are extremely useful, in that they influence how patients think about and interpret the dental experience. That is, some patients will need to be reassured that they "did well" even though they cried a bit or needed a rest break.

There is a second very important aspect to a post-operative discussion. In our experience, even the most skilled clinician at times will not notice that the patient is displeased or upset. In fact, some patients try very hard to mask their feelings. They will allow you to make future appointments for them but will not return once they leave the dental office. We have found that routinely asking all of our patients about the dental experience just completed is an excellent way to identify and ameliorate problems. We ask, "Is there anything I could have done better?" or "Is there anything you would like me to do differently at our next appointment?" Such *debriefing* gives the patient an opportunity to express his feelings and allows us to reinterpret the event and to problem-solve for the next appointment. We believe that everyone in the office or clinic should attempt to debrief some patients. Usually the person who has the most rapport with the patient is delegated to do the debriefing before the patient leaves. This effort will often provide you valuable feedback that you would not ordinarily get. Remember that many of these patients are not assertive and must be "invited" to give you feedback.

SPECIAL CONCERNS FOR DISTRUSTFUL PATIENTS

The best strategy for treating dental fear that is based on distrust is to enhance informational and behavioral control. As with all successful therapy, this must be done within a trusting relationship. Distrustful patients present certain problems, which we discuss below.

Control Issues. Treating a distrustful patient requires you to enhance his sense of personal control. Reassurance: "Everything will be all right—just trust me", especially when you have not yet established a successful working relationship, will have a negative effect and only reinforce patients' distrust.

Of the four major diagnostic categories of fearful patients, distrustful patients are most likely to respond positively to information and explanations. They like things "out in the open," appreciate hearing the "scientific rationale" behind each procedure as it is performed, and often like written detailed written treatment plans. Tell the patient how nice it is to treat someone who is extremely interested in the details of dental care. This is a wonderful opportunity to talk about the scientific basis of dental procedures, evidence for and against a given procedure, and other issues.

Discounting. When you work with distrustful patients it is important not to discount or minimize the complexity of the treatment. For example, when planning treatment, if you are not sure whether or not a tooth requires endodontic treatment it is better to tell distrustful patients that the tooth requires a root canal. If in fact the tooth does require endodonitics, you will be perceived as competent and honest. On the other hand, if you minimized the patient's treatment needs and then told him that, with the tooth being open, it requires a root canal, you will be thought of as either incompetent or dishonest, or both. In addition, for patients with whom you believe you have little rapport, do not minimize the problems of completing treatment. You may even suggest to this patient that he may find dental treatment or working with you a challenge and that he may or may not be successful. In other words, don't over-promise good results to a "doubting Thomas."

Treatment Preferences. As we noted, it is essential to encourage patients to state their views and preferences. This is especially important with distrustful patients. Imagine this scenario:

Patient: Doctor, you know, I know that I have gum problems and these broken teeth in the front of my mouth.

Dentist: I see, do you have any preferences about which problem we work on first?

Patient: Yes, I'm extremely concerned about the way that my front teeth look.

Dentist: I'm glad you told me that because then I would like to recommend that we begin our treatment by trying to remove the decay and to replace missing parts of this front tooth with a cosmetic filling.

Patient: Thank you. I was afraid you would insist on a root canal first. I'm really excited about looking better. That sounds fine to me.

What's different about this approach? Most clinicians have been trained to care for problems in priority order: emergent/acute problems, disease control, and rehabilitation. Cosmetics are usually a lower priority, in part because many of us believe that patients will not return for posterior restorations if we do the anteriors first. In our experience with distrustful patients, failure to attend to their concerns will result in cancellations or "disappearance." We encourage you to do something that shows results early on. Repair anteriors, even if temporarily. Clean anteriors, remove calculus, and stain. If you do this, the patient can experience some success with some simple straightforward procedures, feel good about what the dentist has done, and be much more likely to return.

Safety. Another distrustful but unassertive patient reported feeling dizzy and unable to swallow when the chair was reclined. One of us suggested to the patient that she tell her dentist this so he could adjust the chair. With some encouragement, the patient asserted her feelings. When the dentist adjusted the chair for her there was a palpable sigh of relief and triumph on her face when she knew she had some control.

With this patient, we negotiated a solution to the chair position. We agreed to gradually tilt the chair back, a little bit more each visit, over a series of appointments. Each time we moved it back only as far as she could stand it, then we recorded the chair position in the chart. Soon the problem disappeared and we were back to the original reclined position.

Watching The Dentist. The distrustful patient is often very vigilant, carefully attending to what is going on. Focus this attention and make it useful by giving the patient a mirror. Watching the procedure will let her know what is going on. It makes the treatment concrete and dispels inaccurate perceptions. Encourage the patient's desire to watch and view it as part of his participation in his oral health care. Give him a mirror.

Options. Understanding patient preferences and encouraging these patients to be active in decision making is also essential. Give them as much information as you can and do not let them opt out of decision-making with the "you know best, doctor" ploy. We do not want to place ourselves in the position of persuading or talking this patient into treatment. Written treatment plans and signed consent forms are essential with the distrustful patient. Recall from the discussion on treatment planning in Chapter 4 that it is especially important for distrustful patients to be given treatment options to choose among.

Appointment Scheduling. Patients can express their preferences for the time of day, length of appointment, or intervals between appointments. It is important to allow some flexibility about such things. Imagine these two scenarios:

Receptionist:	Doctor would like you to make an appointment now for preparing your tooth for a crown.
Patient:	That's a stressful procedure for me and I would prefer to have it done in the middle of the day since my husband can come with me.
Receptionist:	I'm sorry, Doctor only does these procedures in the morning.
Patient:	Oh, I see.

Now the alternative:

Receptionist:	Do you have any preferences about when your next appointment is? It will be for your crown.
Patient:	Oh I'm relieved you told me that. I would really like to come in the middle of the day because my husband can drive me.

Receptionist: Good, I'm glad you told me that. Ordinarily, Doctor Good doesn't do these procedures in the middle of the day but I know that he's concerned about making this as easy on you as possible. How about...?

Another problem is the interval between visits. Some patients just want to get treatment over with and wish to come frequently now that they have gotten up their courage to begin treatment. Others may wish to have more time between their appointments. Generally speaking, this timing is unimportant to the success of treatment, and flexibility is rewarded with fewer cancellations. An exception is with a generalized anxiety patient who has a strong tendency to worry. Breaks of three to four weeks between appointments tend to let worry build.

Embarrassment Over Oral Cleanliness. In our experience many fearful patients have poor oral hygiene accentuated by lack of contact with dentistry. They are sensitive to criticism, however benign, and most dental professionals criticize. It is almost as if we prefer that all our patients come to us healthy. It should not be so surprising that many anxious and fearful patients arrive with very poor oral hygiene. Imagine this scenario (our patients do):

Patient: I'm really embarrassed to let you look in my mouth. I haven't been taking very good care of my mouth. (Dental Hygienist looks into mouth.)

Hygienist: You're right, you have some pretty serious problems! How much do you value your oral health?

Perhaps a better approach would have been:

Hygienist: I can see you have an on-going infection in your mouth. I'm glad you came to see us now because it's possible to get it under control, especially if we have your active participation. Later on, with your permission, I would like to teach you some special cleaning skills that you can use in helping control the problem. It is difficult to clean some

> of your teeth because of the way they are set...
> Do you have any questions? ... If you should
> have a question later, please feel free to...

It is important to remember that these patients will take any sign of belittlement as a confirmation that they should put off dental care. They may rationalize avoidance by saying "this dental hygienist doesn't understand my problem" or "this dentist isn't willing to be accommodating." The dentist or hygienist who succeeds with the anxious patient *accepts* the problem and is *flexible* in remediating it.

Self-Help Strategies. The distrustful patient is a great candidate for home care instruction. Being able to control the disease process permits a measure of independence from health care providers that these patients relish. It is a tremendous opportunity for the dentist or staff to praise the patient's progress and support her efforts. As always, a well prepared professional is most effective. For example:

Hygienist: The bacteria that live on your teeth cause the redness and bleeding in your gums. I'd like to apply some food coloring on your teeth and stain these bacterial colonies so they are easier to see. (Demonstrate)

Patient: What do I look for?

Hygienist: See the dark red stains here between your teeth? (Pointing)

Patient: Yes.

Hygienist: Good, this red stuff highlights the bacterial deposits that you need to consistently remove in order to return your gums to health.

We suggest that you keep records such as a plaque map in the chart, and use these records each visit to reinforce progress. Set readily achievable goals and move forward one step at a time. This way you will be able to find something to praise at each appointment. Sincere social reinforcement helps dispel distrust. Consult the part of Chapter 9 on home care instruction for more suggestions.

CONCLUSION

Establishing trust and control are key elements in working with the patient. They are enhanced, in part, by what you say and, more importantly, by specific actions that you take. Information, offering choices, and behavioral control are especially useful with the distrustful patient.

QUESTIONS AND EXERCISES

1. List several specific techniques that can help gain a patient's trust. Write out specific questions and statements that you could say to the patient to begin this process.

2. Cite some specific ways in which dental auxiliaries can set the tone for an open, trusting relationship with patients.

3. Imagine a new patient who seeks care at your office for a mouth that needs extensive restoration and home care. Write out a conversation in which you attempt to project yourself as an interested, concerned person and health care provider.

4. Describe at least one way to facilitate your patient's sense of control from each of the three categories: Informational, Behavioral, Retrospective.

5. Discuss the concept of perceived control over treatment procedures with one of your next patients. Using your own words, ask how much control he feels he actually has. That is, what do you think he can or cannot do? How would you classify it? Ask if he would like more or less control.

SIX

Psychological and Pharmacological Management:

Specific Strategies

- Physical Strategies
- Cognitive Strategies
- Practice Strategies
- Pharmacological Strategies

The Problem: Anticipation and Worry

As we discussed earlier, it is the patient's negative expectations, the active recall of past negative events, influenced by his lack of self efficacy which reactivates fear at subsequent dental appointments. Consequently, in many cases, if no effort is made to have a patient think or feel differently, he will think and feel as he has in the past. Caught up in emotional upset and arousal he will recall almost nothing about his current dental experience. It won't matter if from an objective point of view the present dental experience is painless, or a "good experience." That is why for many fearful patients, experience with a kind, gentle dentist is often *not enough* to make much of a difference in the patient's perceptions about dentistry. Even if the appointment is "painless" or turns out well, what the patient remembers after each visit is that she felt bad, "wiped out," embarrassed, or humiliated, and she doesn't want to return to that situation.

Most fearful patients will benefit from learning and using one or more strategies to control or change their thoughts. The traditional method is to use an anti-anxiety drug such as nitrous oxide or diazepam, a topic we will discuss later in the chapter. But we will first examine two kinds of strategies for inducing relaxation and controlling anxiety: physical and mental relaxation

Research has conclusively shown that anticipation of an event leads to measurable changes in physiological states. As early as 1963, a series of careful studies by Shannon and Isbell made it clear that marked emotional reactions, as measured by urinary cortisol, derive mainly from the anticipation of dental procedures. Shannon and Isbell subjected 258 healthy young men to an injection procedure. Because the men had not been aware that they were scheduled for dental work, their long-term anticipation was held to a minimum. The study involved five experimental treatments: (1) injection of 2 percent lidocaine HCl; (2) injection of 2 percent lidocaine HCl with epinephrine, 1:100,000; (3) injection of 0.9 percent sodium chloride; (4) needle insertion with no injection; (5) a statement that the injection would shortly occur, but no actual injection. In the latter condition, the needle was placed in the subject's mouth but never touched the tissues. This mock injection provided the anticipation condition, a purely psychological procedure.

The results clearly showed that all of the experimental conditions produced significant increases in hydrocortisone in the urine. What is particularly interesting is that the mock injection procedure produced as much hormonal increase as any of the other procedures. This demonstrates that expectation produced the full emotional response. Anticipation of harm is present in each of the physical conditions.

Laboratory experiments by Lazarus and his colleagues (1966) further demonstrate the important role of anticipation. Investigators compared reactions to "suspense" films showing a sequence of

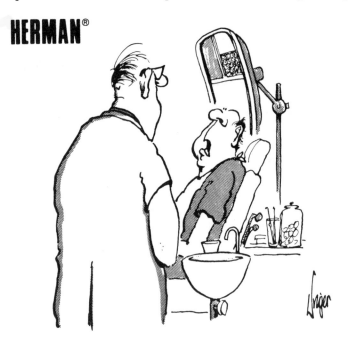

HERMAN®

"Why did your nurse want to know my 'next-of-kin'?"

events leading to an industrial accident with reactions to a "surprise" film they had made by excising the footage leading up to the accident. The autonomic arousal, measured by heart rate and skin conductivity, was greater in the group that watched the suspense film. Moreover, for both films, most of the rise in subjects' autonomic functioning occurred *before* the accident was shown; seeing the accident added comparatively little to the reaction that had occurred during anticipation.

Research has shown that merely telling someone to "relax" is different from relaxation training, which takes concentration and practice. Clum *et al.* (1982) presented evidence that the results are different. Relaxation training is more effective in reducing pain-related distress and the verbal report of pain than are simple instructions to "try and relax" without training.

Using a Patient's Coping Skills

All of us are able to get through stressful situations in our lives. Of course, some of us do better than others. Many of us, for example, feel nervous about speaking in front of an audience. Some have found it useful to imagine thunderous applause to the talk. As we suggested in Chapter 4, it helps to ask a fearful patient, "How do you cope with *other* stressful situations in your life?" Our goal is to uncover coping techniques the person already uses which he can apply in the dental setting.

Coping strategies are often taught as part of weight control, smoking cessation, martial arts, natural childbirth, and stress reduction programs. Among the most common strategies are meditation, auto-hypnosis, relaxation, visual imagery, and deep breathing. They all encourage the person to focus on a comfortable or competing mental image or word phrase (*mantra*) which acts to counter or block out the fear producing thoughts. The patient practices visualizing, or mentally repeating, a coping phrase over and over. Physical relaxation techniques are often used in combination with this approach.

We suggest that you ask anxious patients if they are familiar with any of these techniques. If so, encourage them to apply these skills during treatment, because few patients will know that they can and should be used during dentistry. Your suggestion will come as a welcome relief.

Case Example

Some time ago we saw a 40-year-old man with severe periodontal disease. His dentition was intact but he was at high risk for loss of his teeth. He could not tolerate scaling procedures even when his gums were numb. He worried constantly about being hurt, the sensations, and feeling foolish. The dental hygienist found out that he practiced a martial arts technique that would have helped him relax but had not thought to use it in the dental chair.

She asked the patient to explain what he did.

Patient:	When I begin my exercises, I must concentrate deeply on them. I focus on my breathing. I am still, relaxed, and in deep thought. I can block out noises.
Dental Hygienist:	This is a very valuable technique. If you can practice that skill here, you will find it will compete successfully with the negative thoughts you have been having about dentistry. But it will help you to have a warm-up period before each appointment, here in the operatory. We'll ask you to signal us when you are ready.
Patient:	What if it doesn't work?
Dental Hygienist:	What you will experience, especially the first few times, is that your concentration will be occasionally disturbed by a dental procedure. We will stop, and give you the time to regain your concentration. Each time you refocus it will become easier, and eventually you will find that fewer events "bump" you out of your relaxed state.

We will now examine various strategies patients can use to cope more effectively in the dental environment.

PHYSICAL STRATEGIES: RELAXING THE BODY

Relaxation Breathing

The most important and fundamental relaxation skill which you can teach an anxious patient is fortunately the simplest, and one of the most effective.

Westerners have only recently become aware of the effects of breathing and muscle tone in the role of relaxation. Relaxed patients simply do not feel nearly as much mental or physical discomfort as those who are tense (Thompson, 1977). Thus, it is a good idea to use some simple techniques that will enhance physical relaxation. For centuries, breathing exercises have been integral parts of mental, physical, and spiritual development in the Orient and India. As the West hurries to catch up with the East in understanding and using breath control, it has borrowed heavily from the teachings of Yoga. The underlying goal of all Yoga is to enable a person to control his body and mind through self-discipline.

When an insufficient amount of fresh air reaches someone's lungs, blood is not properly oxygenated. Poorly oxygenated blood contributes to anxiety states, depression, and fatigue and makes stressful situations such as dental treatment harder to cope with (Spreads, 1978). When a patient "white knuckles it" and "holds on for dear life," her physiological arousal is increased and she is much more likely to be "jumpy" and over-reactive, exhibiting startle responses each time she is surprised by a new sound or sensation. Sitting in the chair "waiting to be hurt" also results in the patient's becoming an unreliable reporter of pain and discomfort.

We introduce the concept of relaxation to patients by explaining much of what we have discussed above. For example, we might say,

> I think it's important that I help you find some things *you* can do to make yourself as comfortable as possible during dental treatment. I don't want you to have to rely solely on me to make this a tolerable experience. One of the most important things that you can learn is how to keep yourself as physically relaxed as you can in a difficult situation like this. A simple strategy called paced breathing will help keep you "off the edge" and make you less jumpy.

Begin by asking the patient to slowly fill his lungs. "I want you to slowly take in a *deep* breath to a *slow* count of five, hold for a second, and then to 'sigh' or exhale slowly." Your personal demonstration of this simple technique is useful. Point out to the patient that the muscles are much more relaxed when you are exhaling. Physically guide the patient through four or five very slow breaths. You may find it helpful to place your hand on his shoulder, lifting gently up on the "in" breath and then pushing down when he exhales to help him establish the rhythm. Other patients will find it useful for you to count for them during both exhaling and inhaling. Tell the patient that his eyes can be open or closed, though many find it easier to concentrate with them closed. Request that he continue for two to four minutes. Most anxious patients will become noticeably more comfortable. Patients with elevated heart rates can frequently reduce their BPM 12-20 beats quite rapidly, and you can proceed as soon as their breathing becomes slow and rhythmic.

This exercise is useful for almost every fearful patient. We have found it is often very useful to attach a simple heart rate monitor to the patient during the initial session when learning and practicing this skill. It helps both you and the patient assess one aspect of her arousal and her success in controlling it with basic relaxation strategies. We discuss the use of a heart rate monitor in more in detail in the section on biofeedback.

Another variation of this technique involves focusing on exhalation. Begin by asking the patient to complete two slow and deep breathing cycles, slowly exhaling while counting to five or six. Then, after the third breathing cycle, instruct her not to inhale for as long as possible. When she can no longer restrain breathing, tell her to inhale deeply and to attend to the relief she experienced. Follow this respiratory relief by two slow and deep breathing cycles (Longo, 1984). Repeat for as long as needed. *Most adult fearful patients tend to hold their breath* during dental procedures, especially during injections or after initial placement of the rubber dam. An alert chairside assistant can help patients pace their breathing. You can use similar procedures to pace the breathing of a patient (most often a child) who is likely to hyperventilate.

Try using breathing exercises before and during impressions. Practice the procedure with an empty tray. Time the practice so that the patient learns how long the real impression procedure will last.

When he indicates that it's OK to begin, do the procedure in the same way you rehearsed it. There may still be some anxious behavior. Nonetheless, praise the patient for successful coping, and then let him regain his composure before you proceed. Repeated successful experiences will result in desensitization to dental procedures.

Try this strategy first with a patient you feel comfortable with. We also encourage you to practice these techniques on yourself. Proper breathing is an antidote to stress for staff as well as for patients!

Finally, there is another type of breathing technique is used in situations where pain control is an issue, such as in natural childbirth. It is a paced "panting" type of breathing. In dentistry, it is most appropriately used during those rare emergencies where your ability to achieve adequate anesthesia is limited, and where you have to proceed with treatment.

Muscle Relaxation

Once the patient masters the fundamentals of breathing it is often helpful to take a few additional minutes to focus on muscle relaxation strategies. As every experienced practitioner knows, most anxious patients tend to "brace themselves for the worst." Unfortunately, this reaction makes the problem worse by providing powerful cues which increase the patient's physiological and mental upset. It is crucial that you counter this situation by using a relaxation strategy.

The procedure that has received the most scrutiny is called "progressive relaxation" and was developed by Edmund Jacobson, a Chicago physician, in 1938. The technique is based on the premise that the body responds to anxiety-provoking thoughts and events with muscle tension. This physical tension, in turn, increases the person's subjective experience of anxiety. Muscle relaxation reduces physiological tension and is incompatible with anxiety. The habit of responding with relaxation blocks anxiety; it is impossible to be physically relaxed and psychologically upset at the same time. This technique has produced excellent results in the treatment of many anxiety-implicated problems including insomnia, fatigue, muscle spasm, neck and back pain, stuttering, high blood pressure, and various phobias.

The procedures are simple but require practice to master. We recommend one or two sessions per day, five to ten minutes each, for one to two weeks. After a demonstration and supervised practice, patients can practice at home. Ask them to practice at the same time and place each day and to record their practice sessions in a log. Notations of how they feel before and after each session will help you and them assess progress.

We have used the following set of instructions with our fearful patients. The basic procedure involves tensing specific muscle groups for five to seven seconds, immediately followed by 20 seconds of relaxation. The procedure may be demonstrated and practiced in a dental chair. Four major muscle groups are tensed and relaxed, one at a time. They are:

1. Feet, calves, thighs, buttocks

2. Hands, forearm, and biceps

3. Chest, stomach, and lower back

4. Head, face, throat, and shoulders

We recommend that you first demonstrate the procedure to the patient with his eyes open. A first session will almost always bring some relaxation. We go through the procedure twice, primarily to demonstrate that practice is valuable in enhancing relaxation. With home practice, it will be possible for the patient to relax in the dental chair in just a few minutes. Making an audio tape of the second time through the procedure and providing it to the patient to play at home can be a useful strategy. It is helpful to talk slowly and softly to the patient and to provide suggestions during the relaxation phases.

You could use the following expressions:

Relax and smooth out the muscles ... Let the tension melt away ...

Loose ... limp ... calm ... Feel rested ... calm ... tension gone ...

Here are the instructions and procedure we use:

Find a comfortable position ... and relax. Now clench your

fists, tighten ... tighten. Feel the tension ... Notice the tension in your fist and forearm. Now relax. Feel the looseness. Notice the contrast with the tension. Now bend your elbows and tense your biceps ... as hard as you can. Feel the tautness. Okay, relax, straighten out your arms. Let them hang there loose and limp. Loose and limp, let the relaxation come to you. Feel the difference.

Now let us go to your feet. Curl your toes. Do you feel your calves tense? Good. But don't tense so much that your muscles will cramp. Now relax. Let the tension melt away. Muscles feel loose and limp?

Now we will turn our attention to your neck and shoulders. Lots of tension there. Crunch them up and tighten them ... more ... Okay ... relax. Warm, comfortable, loose and limp. Relaxed. Allow your brow to become smooth again.

Now clench your jaw, biting hard, lips slightly parted, as if you were angry. Relax. Feel the difference? Notice that your jaw is slightly open. This is a natural, relaxed position. The more relaxed your face and mouth are the easier dentistry will be for you. Good ... you are doing fine. Let *all* of your body relax. Enjoy the calm peaceful feeling. Your body is heavy and loose. Relaxed ...

We find it most useful to use rhythmic breathing in coordination with the muscle tightening and relaxation. As the patient inhales, have him tense a specific set of muscles. When he exhales, have him relax the muscles. Suggest looseness in the chest. "Hear the slow hiss and continue relaxing. Let your breathing become slow, free, and gentle. Notice even more tension leaving you and how comfortable you feel."

Being able to relax quickly and effectively is a *skill*. Remember that practice is important, just as it is for any physical activity like learning a new dance step, or proper form for a backhand in tennis. Demonstrate the skill, have the patient practice at home. Encourage the patient to employ the relaxation skills in other stressful situations. When the patient comes in for the next appointment, seat him in the chair a few minutes early to relax and practice his relaxation and breathing exercise before the dental work begins. With practice, tensing and relaxing of the arms and shoulders is usually sufficient to provide a cue to the patient to relax.

The following passages are excerpts from a log one of our patients kept of her practice. You may want to have your patients keep a log like this.

12/1 11:00 P.M.

I was over-tired and it was hard to get to sleep, so I did relaxation breathing, listening to very soft music. My body became very relaxed, and like you said, the breathing takes over. I didn't even realize I was breathing. Soon the breathing became almost trance like. It is an unusual feeling, it seems like someone else is controlling my breathing. As I went along further it seemed like my breathing slowed down considerably. I stopped after 5 minutes. Got to sleep sooner than I normally would.

12/2 4:30 P.M.

Our computer system at work went down and we lost all the work that was keyed in since 11:00 A.M., and I was working with our engineer over the phone to get the system up. This was very upsetting because I knew that I would have to work Saturday to make up the work and I really had my heart set on going to the mountains. I was upset and under a lot of stress. During my lunch at 12:30 I laid down and did the muscle and breathing exercises which helped a lot. When my lunch was through I went back to work feeling better and ready to tackle the work.

12/4 2:00 P.M.

Muscle tensing and relaxing really help but I have a way where I focus completely on various parts of my body and cause them to relax. I usually start from my feet and up and out to my hands.

12/5 4:00 P.M.

Having extremely bad menstrual cramps so I laid down. I decided to do the relaxation and breathing. It helped.

12/8

I have been doing the exercises twice daily but the writing is not so regular. One of the easiest and most relaxing times is before I go to sleep. Today wasn't very successful.

12/9

A day off from work for me. Shopped all day so I was ready for some relaxation. Started and I fell asleep.

There are many books written for the general public on self-taught stress reduction and relaxation techniques. For those who would like more information, examine *Relaxation Dynamics: A cognitive-behavioral approach*, by J.C. Smith (Champaign, Illinois, Research Press, 1989).

Physiological Monitoring: Biofeedback

Within Wolpe's technique is the essence of a far-reaching idea—the view that man may acquire voluntary control over a variety of physiological functions, and, in doing so, alter his psychological state. This idea has its roots in eastern disciplines such as Yoga and Zen. More recently western science and therapies such as progressive relaxation and autogenic training have validated the idea.

Three interesting developments may extend the range and power of this approach: the rapid growth and proliferation of inexpensive electronic instrumentation; research involving events that were previously difficult to measure; and the attempt to identify psychophysiological pathways or feedback loops. Measuring a physiological event electronically and converting the electronic signal to visual, auditory, or other comprehensible feedback permits continuous awareness of a physiological state. This is the essence of biofeedback. A patient's awareness of physiological events she had not previously attended to gives her voluntary control over physiological functions, many of which were once considered totally involuntary. For example, we know that an individual can learn to lower blood pressure with biofeedback training.

These developments have led to advances in research and treatment primarily in stress-related disorders. The medical literature reports widespread use of biofeedback in the treatment of tension and migraine headache, muscle pains, irritable bowel syndrome, and insomnia. The dental literature reports the success of this approach in treating myofacial pain-dysfunction syndrome, clenching, and bruxism (Flor & Birbaumer, 1993).

Biofeedback has been used to treat dental fear. Hirschman and colleagues (1980, 1982) have shown that various biofeedback procedures can be useful in managing dental fear. Using electromyographic (EMG) feedback, Hirschman (1980) in a single brief session trained dental patients to decrease muscle activity in the forearm. Highly anxious patients who received biofeedback were less anxious during treatment and reported that their restorative dental treatment was less stressful than they had anticipated. Highly anxious control group patients, on the other hand, showed increases in anxiety and reported that procedures were more stressful than they had anticipated. Oliver and Hirschman (1982) reported that subjects with severe dental anxiety exposed to heart rate biofeedback reported less unpleasantness and showed lower heart rates as they viewed videotapes of stressful dental procedures than did similar subjects provided with relaxation instructions or those in a control situation.

We have found that monitoring heart rate is particularly useful for patients in three situations. First, some patients recognize (or believe) that their heart beats wildly when they are fearful. Once they are taught basic physical relaxation skills, we hook them up to a heart rate monitor and use it to provide feedback on how well they are implementing their relaxation strategies. Patients whose hearts respond to fear find that they can effectively lower their heart rate. In fact, we often make lowering their heart rate a *condition* for proceeding with treatment. For example, we might say: "Jane, when you first sat down your resting heart rate was 80 BPM. Now that we are ready for the injection it is almost 100! I want you to take a couple of minutes to practice your breathing techniques and relax. As soon as you get it back down, I'll proceed with the injection."

Heart rate monitoring is also useful for patients who do not recognize their own anxiety—that is, for the patient who whose heart is pounding madly away but is unaware of it. We point out what we observe and then explain the reason that it is important to get the heartbeat back into a more normal range.

Third, biofeedback can be very helpful with patients who are fearful of a medical catastrophe: those who believe their bodies may "go out of control" during dental treatment. Patients who fear adverse medical events are discussed in more detail in Chapter 8.

Simple but accurate heart rate monitors can be purchased in any athletic and exercise equipment store. We have found that monitors which use an ear clip, rather than those which attach on the finger, are easier to use in the dental setting. Prices range from $50 to $100.

Note: As described in Chapter 8, there is a small percentage of patients, some of whom have a history of agoraphobia, who actually become more fearful when they try to relax or are given feedback on their heart rate. Consequently, it is useful to question patients about their experiences with relation training.

COGNITIVE STRATEGIES: RELAXING THE MIND

We have examined physical (muscle and breathing) relaxation strategies. We will now turn our attention to the other half of the coping equation: What the patient thinks and feels. As we mentioned above, what the patient anticipates, thinks, or worries about is crucial in determining what the patient experiences, no matter what the objective nature of the situation is. In this section we will examine how you can help the patient alter her fearful thoughts. All of us use one or more of these strategies. Otherwise we couldn't deal with the stresses of modern life!

However, many people, and most fearful patients, tend to believe that their feelings and thoughts "just happen," and that there is little that can be done about them because, "I just feel that way." But, psychological research of the last two decades has shown that cognitions are easily changed and influenced by what is happening, or what we expect to happen. We also have learned that feelings are triggered by thoughts, even if they occur so quickly that we are unaware of thinking them. What does this have to do with treating fearful patients?

In essence, the fearful patient anticipates in advance, sometimes a few seconds, sometimes for a few weeks, a dreadful event. His mind is "filled" or focused on fear which leads to both emotional and physiological arousal and discomfort. If we do not act to intervene, if we do not help the patient think or feel differently, *there is no reason to expect* her to notice that the experience is not as bad as she expected.

The first scientifically based approach to this problem was Behavioral Therapy. During the 1960's a number of techniques known as Flooding, Implosion, and Graduated Exposure were researched extensively. Investigators found that if a fearful person were placed in a controlled situation with the feared stimulus, and exposed to it *long* enough, his fear would eventually extinguish. Little attention was paid to the patient's thoughts or feelings. It was found that the individual would gradually "learn" that he was "safe" and that there was nothing to fear. Although treatment was successful, it had to be carefully controlled and repeated often.

However, beginning in the late 1970s a new approach was developed known as Cognitive Behavioral Therapy. It acknowledges that what the patient thinks is important and that the process of overcoming fear is made more efficient if we work with the patient's thought processes in the context of repeated exposures. The patient's task is straightforward: to find a strategy to keep his thoughts from focusing entirely on his worries about the feared situation. In the Dental Fears Research Clinic we tell our patients that these thoughts are "mental videotapes" of dental horror movies. Difficult strategies can change or "unplug" these old tapes. Below we discuss the most common approaches. You must help the patient select and practice a strategy which appears to best fit his personality.

Altering Expectations: Redefining Success and Offering Praise

Our work with fearful persons has led us to realize that they need small methodical steps to overcome their fears. However, many people want a "magic bullet" or quick solution. That is why so many patients ask to "be knocked out" when they come to see us. Do not allow patient pressure for an unrealistically quick solution to alter *your* behavior.

Because of their tendency to seek a quick solution, and because they think that they cannot cope, patients need praise at each step of treatment. Consider the following case. We treated a patient in the Dental Fears Research Clinic who had severe periodontal disease. The treatment involved repeated root planing and curettage under local anesthetic. We taught the patient a relaxation exercise that he practiced for a week before his first injection and treatment. The dental hygienist spent several minutes having the patient practice the relaxation procedure and then administered an infiltration injection.

Afterwards the following occurred:

Patient: Whew! I'm glad that's over. I *still* felt anxious during the injection.

Hygienist: I expected that you would, but you managed very well.

Patient: Yes, but I felt embarrassed when you had to keep reminding me to breathe.

Hygienist: Overcoming these fears takes time and patience. You did great! I'm pleased with your progress. Practicing the relaxation exercises last week really paid off. Shall we proceed?

The scaling was then carried out successfully. We must clearly let patients know that they are making progress, or were successful in their efforts.

At first some patients do not easily accept praise. The anxious patient may continue to discount his progress and still want a quick solution. He may need several visits to overcome his doubts of self-efficacy or his feelings of being unable to master the coping. Do not promise complete success, such as finishing a feared procedure by a certain appointment, or a total reduction of fears. In doing this, you avoid creating a situation where the patient may feel like a failure. With frequent praise and repeated attempts, patients will master the skills they need *and* feel good about themselves. Litt (1993) reported that patients undergoing third molar extractions experienced significantly lower preoperative anxiety when given relaxation and self-efficacy coping strategies. No matter how small the step forward, we all need feedback about our performance in order to improve. Providing coping strategies and positive "strokes" really work.

On the other hand, some patients are completely preoccupied with their imminent or actual discomfort. Initially, they are unwilling to focus on anything else; all reports are negative. Helping these patients recognize and verbalize neutral or positive perceptions is crucial.

Fordyce (1976) presents techniques for chronic pain patients which are useful for the dental patient. After you establish rapport, Fordyce recommends that you redirect the patient's attention to desired perceptions and verbalizations and ignore his maladaptive focus on discomfort. Thus, we reinforce patients' attention to positive or neutral verbalizations and praise their positive self-reports of progress. We give less reinforcement for negative comments. For example, a debriefing after a session might proceed like this:

Dentist: How did it go? Anything I could have done better?

Patient: Well … it was terrible! You said you wouldn't hurt me, but when you put on the rubber dam you pinched me twice.

Dentist: OK, I am glad you told me that, but I wish you had told me at the time. Don't let negative thoughts store up; let me know as soon as they happen. What went right about the appointment?

Altering Expectations: Redefining the Experience

Expectations have the dual effect of facilitating the entry of certain stimuli and inhibiting others. When more than one occurs at the same time, the one we are prepared for has an advantage and is the one we are most likely to notice. Once our response is under way, the other responses are blocked. This is true not only for pain but also for other thoughts and sensations.

A patient's expectation is capable of influencing whether and how she experiences sensations. Anticipation of what is to follow will itself influence the experience. In a study of experimentally induced pain (Chaves & Barber, 1974), subjects who were led by researchers to expect a reduction in pain compared to their initial trial, but who were not provided with a coping strategy, in fact reported a significant reduction in pain. Dworkin and colleagues found that pain tolerance was reduced by increasing subjects' expectations of *heightened* bodily sensations when nitrous oxide was administered (Dworkin et al., 1983). Clinically, there is evidence that expectation can influence positive treatment outcomes. Clinicians communicate expectations both verbally and nonverbally; this may be the central reason for the success of a particular clinical technique.

An example of how expectation affects treatment is seen in the use of audioanalgesia. Gardner and Licklider (1959) and Gardner, Licklider, and Weisz (1960) investigated the effectiveness of white noise and music in suppressing dental pain. They reported that music promotes relaxation and that white noise directly suppresses pain. It was not long before other clinicians were using this technique but with mixed results. As Melzack (1973) described it, some dentists and patients achieved dramatic results. With others, it did not work at all. Many dentists quickly became disillusioned. In a controlled laboratory study, Melzack, Weisz, and Sprague (1963) demonstrated that white noise did not abolish the pain of putting a hand in an ice bucket for five minutes (the cold pressor test). They compared three groups of subjects. Group 1 received strong white noise and music but no suggestion about the purpose of stimulation. Group 2 received strong white noise and music along with a suggestion of its effectiveness for reducing pain. Group 3 received suggestion but only a low-frequency control hum. Each group served as its own control, having received ice bucket pain without any sound before and after the experimental condition. In Group 2 (noise, music, and suggestion), there was a substantial increase in how long the subjects could keep their hands in the bucket, but in Group 1 (noise and music) and Group 3 (control), there was not. Expectations of effectiveness are critical.

Of the four diagnostic types of fearful patients we have identified, it is the patient with generalized anxiety who most needs help in altering her beliefs about her ability to cope. People in this group are also most likely to have unrealistically high expectations about themselves and how they should feel about dental care. They are likely to feel that they are "failing" if the relaxation strategies they try do not produce "total relaxation." Imagine the following conversation:

Dentist: On a scale of 1–10 with 10 the worst, how anxious do you usually feel during an injection?

Patient: Oh, a 10 for sure!

Dentist: Okay. Right now I want you to take a couple of minutes to do your relaxation exercises that you have been practicing at home. *(patient breathes)* How do you feel now?

Patient: About a 7. I guess its not working very well.

Dentist: No no. That's a big change. The goal is not to make you fearless, but to take getting a shot out of the terrifying category and make it into something which may still be difficult, but tolerable. Take another couple of minutes and see if you can relax even further before we proceed.

Fortunately, patients who worry and anticipate are also the most open to suggestion, reassurance, and the authority of the health professional. They tend to respond readily to enthusiasm, smiles, and praise, and they accept and appreciate your concern. As suggested in the model of self-efficacy in Chapter 2, this patient *wants* to be cooperative; what he lacks is a belief that what he can do will be effective, or that what he does is "good" enough. He sets unrealistically high standards for himself, which he repeatedly fails to meet. These patients have very high avoidance gradients just before visits and are the most likely to cancel and not respond to appointment confirmation calls. As noted above, when you begin to work with this type of patient, it is useful to start by helping him set both realistic expectations and reasonable definitions of success and coping.

Distraction

Distraction is the cognitive coping strategy which is most familiar to dental care providers and is probably the easiest of the cognitive techniques to implement.

Researchers have found that electronic games, television, and taped relaxation instruction can control high levels of fear in both dental and medical patients. For example, watching TV (Venham, 1977), and playing video Ping-Pong (Corah *et al.*, 1979a) have been used as distraction techniques during drilling. The experimental work of Corah and associates indicates that a distraction strategy is efficacious in comparison to control strategies. Their work assessing the effect of tape recorded relaxation instructions (Corah *et al.*, 1979a,b, 1981) shows that a repetitive set of relaxation instructions played 3 to 4 minutes before anesthesia, and continued until the procedure was completed, was effective in alleviating anxiety. This strategy relies heavily on distraction: that is, diverting attention from the dental procedure to the tape or to various muscle groups. The key is asking the patient to try to choose an *engaging* activity.

For some patients, it is difficult *not* to focus on what they fear *might* happen. Learning how to alter one's focus of attention is a slow, incremental process. Thus, providing distracters may be useful. For example, airlines have always tried to create a distracting environment in flight. Attractive and attentive personnel, alcohol, hot meals, multichannel stereo music, movies, and magazines are all part of a successful technique which helps prevent travelers, many of whom are anxious about flying, from thinking about being encased in a fragile aluminum and plastic tube, 35,000 feet above the ground. Some of the successful distraction techniques in the dental office can be built right into the environment. Decorating offices with nontraditional decor and using space to eliminate sights, sounds, and smells traditionally associated with dentists' offices is a widely used and helpful strategy. In fact, dentists have traditionally used the technique of diverting attention to facilitate child management. Talking to a child about his favorite animal while the child is being examined is an example of this technique. Such techniques can be equally successful with the adult patient.

Music is one of the easiest distraction techniques to use. With portable tape and CD players so inexpensive, we encourage many patients to bring CDs or tapes of music, books, or comedy they find engaging. Let the patient control the volume. That way he can use it to drown out noises, such as the drill or highspeed vacuum. Encourage the patient to obtain a tape or CD he would enjoy, but has not yet heard. New music tends to be more distracting than old favorites.

However, there are limitations to the effectiveness of distraction. The more intense the patient's fear, and the stronger his tendency to anticipate and worry, the less likely distraction will work, especially during the initial appointments. In such cases even if the patient is receptive to using distraction, it may not reduce the fear to an acceptable level during injections or drilling. Structured time is very

useful with distraction (see Chapter 8). Many patients can successfully distract themselves for a series of short intervals. With moder-
ately fearful patients distraction may be very effective but there will
still be times when the patient's fears will resurface and disrupt his
relaxation efforts. Patients should routinely be counseled to expect
that such interruptions are normal and do not indicate that they, or
the strategy, is failing. They should be allowed to rest briefly and
then instructed to return attention to the distracter. Finally, distraction is not appropriate for every patient. Some people, especially
those who are information oriented or somewhat distrustful, dislike
this technique. For these patients a more active, participatory coping
strategy is appropriate.

Guided Imagery

Guided imagery is similar to distraction. You and the patient agree
upon a particular mental image. For example, a patient may choose
taking a walk by the ocean, spending time with his grandchild,
playing a game of basketball, or digging in the garden as the image
he wishes to think about. You deliberately lead the patient on the
pleasant, engaging mental fantasy by calling up certain images. For
example:

Dentist: OK. I am ready to begin with the topical followed
          by an injection. I want you to take a few deep
          breaths to physically relax. I want you to close your
          eyes and use your imagination to create a mental
          image of all the sights, sounds, smells and
          sensations of the beach walk we discussed before.
          I'll suggest a few images to help you focus. Ready?

Patient: Ready to give it a try at least.

Dentist: Picture yourself walking along the shore looking
          out at the waves rolling in. Hear the sound of the
          restless waves ... Look up at the sky and see those
          white puffy clouds slowly drifting high above past
          the sun ... Feel the sand crunch between your toes
          as you walk ... Feel the sun and wind on your
          face...

The idea is to talk in a slow relaxed manner, trying to get the patient to engage as many senses and memories as possible so that he can get through a particularly difficult procedure.

Focusing Attention

Attention itself exerts considerable influence on what we experience as dental patients. We are all capable of focusing our attention on certain kinds of incoming sensory information, to the exclusion of others. Kanfer and Goldfoot (1966) showed that attention influenced pain tolerance in the test described earlier involving keeping a hand in an ice bucket. Subjects distracted by viewing slides or watching a clock were able to keep their hands in the ice the longest. This classic study confirmed the common sense notion that attention-demanding stimuli can function as a distraction and diminish pain perception.

The selective focusing of attention is itself subject to influence by previous experience. Students "turn off" a lecturer, and workers on the assembly line think of after-work activities to get through the day. Such selectivity of attention results in greater comfort and allows us to avoid much of an aversive experience. Because of its survival value, we repeat it in future situations. Many of us have learned, through stress reduction classes, auto-hypnosis, meditation, or an Asian martial art, to enter into a focused mental state.

Other patients have learned that it is very helpful to engage in prayer or mentally recite a particular Psalm while undergoing certain procedures. Self-employed people often can use chair time to think through a particularly vexing business problem. Still others will be familiar with meditation techniques which are designed to empty the mind of *all* thought. What these procedures have in common is that they are internally generated attention focusing strategies. These techniques work best with people who know that they can concentrate and who routinely do it in other situations.

Practice is necessary. As is the case with physical relaxation, these strategies become more automatic as they are practiced. The patient learns that he is able to focus his attention and thoughts as he wishes. The goal of practice is to teach the patient to gain some control over his cognitive processes and direct them in two ways. The first task is to refrain from thinking about what *might* happen, by focusing his thoughts somewhere else. Researchers (Chaves & Brown, 1978) have found that simply eliminating catastrophic thoughts is sufficient by itself as a coping skill.

The second is to focus attention on what is actually happening moment to moment during dental treatment. For example, a patient who is holding her breath, gripping the chair tightly, and bracing herself for the worst is (unless you are hurting her), *anticipating* disaster. She is spending all her mental energy remembering past experiences or fearing what *might* happen. You need to help her focus on distracting thoughts, *or* pay closer attention to her actual experience.

One way dental care providers have traditionally accomplished this is to give the patient a mirror so that she can really see what is going on. The strategy we discussed earlier of having the patient give us a report on a 1-10 scale of "how painful," "how bad" it was is another way to anchor the patient's perception on what is actually going on. Another technique is to have the patient identify a simple phrase which helps him focus. For example, we sometimes have patients mentally repeat over and over phrases something like this: "I'm scared but nothing bad (painful) is happening to me right now. If it stays this way I'll be OK." This "broken record" strategy can help keep the patient whose thoughts tend to "run away" focused on her actual experience, which is not nearly as painful or scary as the dental horror movie that plays unbidden in her mind.

Thought Stopping

Another variant of cognitive coping is thought stopping. A basic step is for the patient to identify and imagine the stressful thoughts that most often frighten him. After that, he can practice the technique, which is best to do at home.

Ask the patient to ruminate on the stressful thought and then to shout "Stop!" When his shouts have eliminated the thought on several occasions, the patient should try to interrupt the thought with "stop" or whatever word is needed, but in a normal voice. Subsequent sessions will allow him to control the thought with the command verbalized in a whisper. The goal of the process is to use a sub-vocal command to oneself; that is, to imagine hearing "stop!" shouted within one's mind.

The last step of the procedure involves *thought substitution,* the "broken record" technique discussed above. Instruct the patient to replace the stressful thought with a positive self-statement that he has used before, or help him make up messages to use. Some messages our patients have used successfully are: "You have lots of skills you can use." "Just remember to keep active and do what you have to do," and "Don't worry; worrying won't help."

Patients can do much of the thought-stopping procedure at home, and they should practice at least twice a week. Their logs should record all activities. Little time is required to explain these procedures and to review patient logs and progress.

Failure at initial attempts should not discourage you or your patient, because the most stressful thoughts may be difficult to control. Select a less frightening or intense thought to work on while developing proficiency with the technique. Point out that this technique takes time. The thought will return, and the patient will have to eliminate or interrupt it again and again. He will have to stifle each thought as it begins, and substitute alternative thoughts. Success rarely occurs without some practice.

One last consideration: if "Stop!" or another sub-vocalization is inadequate, you might recommend that the patient keep a rubber band unobtrusively around his wrist. When the stressful thought occurs, have the patient snap it. Such behaviors reinforce the sub-vocalization. For further reading, consult *Anxiety and Stress Disorders: Cognitive-Behavioral Assessment and Treatment,* Larry Michelson and L. Michael Ascher, Editors (Guilford Press, 1987).

PRACTICE STRATEGIES

We have now discussed the two types of relaxation strategies: physical and mental. As we noted, in some cases the patient may be familiar with one or more strategies and simply has to be encouraged to use them during dental treatment. In other cases it will be up to you to help select a strategy and then teach it to the patient. We have found that most fearful patients do better if they use both a physical and cognitive coping strategy at first.

However, with many highly fearful patients it will not be enough to try, for the first time, a control or coping strategy during actual treatment. The patient will be too terrified, too concerned about failure, too timid, or have too much performance anxiety to be successful. For example, you may have shown her how to use the suction device to enhance her sense of control, or discussed a signaling technique to use when she needs a break to catch her breath. However, many patients have a "white coat phobia" and are too timid to implement the strategy for fear of offending you. Embarrassed by their fear, they don't want to "bother" you. Similarly, while a patient may have briefly practiced deep breathing or identified a cognitive strategy to use during the injection, his fear during the actual event may be so strong that he can't pay any attention to it. Some patients need to be incrementally exposed to what is feared. Others need some practice "lessons," "rehearsals," or "dry runs" *before* the procedure in order to become familiar with what will happen *and*, most importantly, to practice their new coping response in the feared situation, but where there is no pressure.

Graduated Exposure and its Variants

There is considerable evidence from the psychological literature that the most effective treatment of a wide variety of fears involves the controlled exposure of patients to what is feared (see Rachman, S.J., *Fear and Courage*, 2nd ed, New York: Freeman, 1990). Graduated, controlled exposure should be the guiding principle in treating patients who have a simple dental phobia and do not have additional psychopathology. The term *graduated* refers to the gradual, step-by-step nature of this approach in which procedures that the patient believes to be easier precede those that she finds more difficult. It is important to emphasize that the patient controls not only the order of procedures she faces but also the duration of the exposure and other variables, such as chair positioning and who is in the operatory at the time of the exposure. In order to determine the order of the exposures, the clinician must know what the patient fears and the extent of the fear. Exposures are incremental, as noted, from least to most feared. After repeated, positive experiences, guided by the patient's responses, fear-related behaviors begin to disappear.

During the use of this procedure the clinician may provide considerable information to the patient about the tools and procedures of dental treatment. For example, in "walking through" the steps involved in a root canal, explanations of the steps involved, their purpose, and how long each can be expected to last all help provide informational control to the patient. You might think of exposure as "tell-show-do" for adults.

Rehearsals

A rehearsal is an opportunity for the patient to practice coping while he is exposed to a *simulated procedure* or part of a procedure. First, the patient demonstrates his ability to cope while in the dental chair. Next, he is exposed to stimuli that are like the feared ones. For example, a patient afraid of an intraoral injection will be exposed to a simulated injection, initially with the cap on. When the patient demonstrates adequate coping to this stimulus, he will be exposed to a simulated injection with the cap off. We recommend multiple exposures at each step for all patients.

Rehearsals are used in countless other activities which are considered somewhat difficult or scary and which require the learner to use skills. For example, scuba diving is most often taught in a shallow, warm, well lighted swimming pool where all the conditions are controlled. Similarly, learning to drive, acting in school plays, and parachuting all use the principle of practice in low-pressure, non-threatening situations. As we mentioned at the beginning of this section, repeated exposure to the feared situation where nothing traumatic happens to the patient is, by itself, a proven method for reducing his fears. Practice sessions for a fearful dental patient can be among your most effective and efficient fear reduction strategies, especially when the patient uses some type of physical and cognitive strategy in conjunction with the exposure. This helps make him an active participant in the process of overcoming the fear, rather than a passive bystander.

Patient progress is assessed by his own self-report and by your monitoring of his heart rate. If the patient rates his upset at 3 or less on a 10-point scale, where 10 is extreme upset and 1 is no upset, and his heart rate is stable and approximates a resting heart rate, the rehearsal is having the desired effect. Subsequently, the patient is told that if he signals agreement during the initial fifteen seconds of a rehearsal with the cap off, an actual injection will take place. Patients reaching this stage are told that this is a "dress rehearsal."

The line between a rehearsal and the procedure itself thus becomes rather thin. Rehearsals continue until the patient signals readiness to receive the injection; the delivery of the anesthetic is often anti-climactic. After this is accomplished, the patient is offered the opportunity to precede actual treatment with a rehearsal or "dress rehearsal" or no rehearsal at all.

Case Example: Substituting Behaviors During Rehearsals for a Patient Fearful of Injections

We recently treated a patient whose story allows us to demonstrate how to put these strategies together. This patient had a long history of intense fear of medical and dental injections. She had resisted injections by biting the dentist, grabbing the syringe, or bolting from the chair. Her last visit to the dentist was five years before our treatment began. Injection was the only dental procedure she feared. She was a competent person who ran her own business in addition to caring for her own family. Paradoxically, sewing machine needles, which routinely caused her injury in her business, did not upset her at all. She tolerated scaling and drilling of a non-vital tooth without anesthetic quite well during her initial three appointments. There were no problems and we got to know her well.

After the initial visits, she agreed to try to solve the anesthetic problem. The steps in desensitizing her were:

1. Presenting the mind-body-pain model

2. Using the tell-show-do model

3. Substituting a coping response for a panic response.

4. Practice rehearsals

The approach involved teaching a coping response and rehearsals. To see how she would actually react, at the first appointment we told the patient we would rehearse by bringing the syringe to her mouth (with the COVER on the needle). Everything went fine as the topical was placed but when the syringe came near, her arm and shoulder muscles tensed. After this, her heart rate increased and she reported feeling panicky.

We asked the patient to rest for a few minutes and then indicate when we could try a second rehearsal. This time we asked her to practice tensing the masseter, clenching, and then to sigh deeply. When she sighed, the masseter relaxed. So when her lip was re-tracted and the dentist placed the syringe this time (again with the COVER in place), he told her to sigh at the first sign of muscle tension. The patient still tensed her muscles a little but did not reach for the syringe, turn away, or show any of the previous interfering behaviors. We praised her for her effort. After resting, she practiced the clenching-relaxing behavior again, when she indicated she was ready.

The analogy we used in explaining the need for this practice was this: "We want your desired reaction to be automatic, just like putting on the car brakes when you see a red traffic light. The more you practice relaxing (or driving), the more automatic it becomes when you are aware that you are getting upset." In this way, the patient gains control over the procedure.

On the third try, the patient successfully allowed the trial to proceed without any resistance, all the while breathing deeply. Again we praised her for her success. At the end of the appointment she was given homework: she would regularly practice imagining the syringe and using the clenching-relaxing exercise before the second appointment.

At the second appointment, after two "cap off" rehearsals, we administered the injection successfully. In less than two hours, a seemingly insurmountable problem was solved and the patient went on to be a highly cooperative and satisfactory participant in dental care.

Systematic Desensitization

For some patients, straightforward rehearsals are not enough. When patients are extremely fearful and indicate that they have very little ability to cope, a more rigorous procedure, systematic desensitiza-tion, is necessary. Very often patients with other psychiatric dis-orders besides simple dental phobia benefit from the use of this procedure.

Wolpe's (1958) systematic desensitization was one of the most encouraging developments in psychology in the last generation. In essence, this technique involves substituting a relaxation response for an anxiety response. Feared stimuli are presented gradually, with the least feared stimulus presented first.

This method of treatment has a long and successful history. Mary Cover Jones (1924) first reported using the procedure to treat a child who was very afraid of rabbits. She gradually moved the feared object closer and closer to the child while the child was preoccupied eating a favorite food. The strategy of substituting a non-fearful for a fearful response was capitalized upon by Joseph Wolpe who used a simplified version of Jacobson's progressive relaxation training as the non-fearful response. Wolpe's technique included generating a hierarchy of fear-producing situations for each patient, specific to the particular fear. The patient is taught to relax and then visualize a scene from the low-fear end of the hierarchy. While maintaining the relaxed state, the patient systematically progresses through all items in the hierarchy. After this, patients are able to calmly face the previously frightening situations.

Wolpe's method, presented in *Psychotherapy by Reciprocal Inhibition* (1958), has had considerable success. It has been applied to a wide range of fears, and variations in the technique have been reported. There is evidence, for example, that exposure to real stimuli (*in vivo* desensitization) has succeeded after imaginal desensitization has failed. In our experience, for fearful dental patients, the *in vivo* treatment appears to be as successful as it is with other monosymptomatic phobias (Yates, 1970). Moreover, we recommend this procedure instead of graduated exposure or rehearsals with patients who have additional psychopathology.

Treating dental fear with systematic desensitization can be traced to the work of Gale and Ayer in 1969. Since then, many case histories illustrating various desensitization techniques have been reported in the literature (e.g., Klepac, 1975). Recent innovative research has used these techniques with groups of fearful patients (Moore & Brodsgaard, 1994).

Case Example

An example of a problem we solved using *in vivo* desensitization involved gagging and fear of choking. The patient was referred by her dentist because she was unable to tolerate treatment of an upper second molar with dental caries. Attempts to obtain a periapical radiograph had failed. The dentist sent along only a panoramic film.

We used a classical systematic desensitization technique to allow her to vividly recreate the sensation of gagging outside the dental chair. Thus, we decided to first recreate the sensation and teach the patient an alternative to panic. In this case, relaxation (and deep breathing) was the preferred response since gagging is caused by muscle tension. As the patient was able to imagine and relax, we moved to the clinic in a series of small graduated steps.

We began working in the anterior region. We had the patient place her finger behind the lower anteriors while she practiced her relaxation skills. With practice, much of it at home, she was quickly able to rest her finger against the upper and lower second molars. We then began having the patient work with a radiograph. Over the next few weeks the patient again practiced at home, coming in for brief, weekly checks on her progress. We then were able to obtain a full mouth series of films.

Sample Dental Fear Hierarchy (Gagging)

Imagine:

- Making an appointment
- Going to the dental office
- Sitting in the waiting room
- Entering the operatory
- Sitting in the chair
- An X-ray tab

Practice:

- Handling tab
- Placing finger at location radiograph to be taken
- Placing tab in mouth and removing
- Placing tab, holding for 8 seconds, breathing twice
- Hygienist placing tab
- Patient holding tab while radiograph is taken

We used the same approach with the rubber dam. Repeated practice at each location, anterior to posterior, produced awareness and mastery. Constant praise, and lots of feedback (e.g., telling her the length of time the rubber dam was on) was very helpful. Again, the speed of exposure depends on the progress the patient is making. There is no way to know in advance whether the treatment will take one or two or even six or seven sessions.

RETURN OF FEAR

While we may be very effective in helping patients remain comfortable during dental procedures they fear, these experiences may not be sufficient to eliminate future dental avoidance and fearful behaviors. Reduction of fear is not always permanent and may return in unexpected ways. A patient may be very successful in overcoming a dental fear and receive a limited amount of needed dental treatment within a period of a month or so. Six months to a year later, when faced with additional dental treatment, he experiences a return of fear and may even delay or avoid treatment. Why does this occur?

The research literature indicates that fear returns more often when the individual does not regularly face the fearful stimuli. The larger the interval between successful fear-reduction experiences and subsequent experiences, the greater the probability of return of fear. This suggests that when patients have a hiatus in the care they receive we should expect and *they should be told to expect* a return of fear. That is why it is more difficult to completely overcome a fear of dental treatment than, say, driving freeways, where the individual has the chance to "practice" frequently. More importantly, this suggests that we should actually plan to keep the patient's intervals between visits and treatments as short as possible.

The research literature also suggests that patients with more exposures will have more success in avoiding return of fear. Providing more than a minimal number of positive experiences will help prevent return of fear.

Independent of their fear treatment experiences, some patients are at greater risk for return of fear. Patients who have a very high heart rate (120 BPM), especially at the start of treatment, are likely to have fear return. In the interval between treatment of fear and subsequent dental experience, being depressed or having an unrelated aversive or fearful experience also appear to trigger return of fear. Finally, patients who are generally anxious, and who worry about many situations in life, appear to have more reoccurances of fear than those who are distrustful or fearful of specific procedures.

When fear does return it is easily treated. It is not necessary to begin at Square One for these patients. The fear that returns may be reduced to manageable levels or entirely eliminated if you and the patient review coping skills and the control mechanisms of choice and if you then provide additional graduated exposures. Opportunities to practice and refamiliarize him with the dental environment will likely result in success.

PHARMACOLOGICAL MANAGEMENT: SPECIFIC STRATEGIES

Psychological versus Pharmacological Management

Many clinicians believe that they must choose between two quite different modes of therapy for the fearful patient: either drugs, such as preoperative oral diazepam, or behavioral treatment, such as training in stress management. However, clinicians are continually influencing patient expectations and behaviors. Thus, even when they use sedative hypnotic agents, their patient preparation will influence the dose of the drug used, the effectiveness of the strategy, and the probability of paradoxical responses and side effects. We strongly recommend preparation for every patient when you plan pharmacologically based fear interventions.

In an experiment involving extremely fearful patients with a long history of avoiding dentistry and extensive dental need, Berggren (1984) randomly assigned subjects to either behavioral treatments and graduated exposure to dentistry, such as is recommended in this book, or general anesthesia to accomplish needed dental care. After initial treatment the patients were given the opportunity to receive regular care in community practices. The community dentists were given information about their patients' previous problems and suggestions for follow-up treatment. The long-term results demonstrate clearly the superiority of the behavioral approach: many of the patients who received general anesthesia-based treatment failed to establish relationships with community dentists while most of those in the alternative condition did establish a base in the community that they maintained. This is not a criticism of drug oriented treatment *per se*; rather, it points up the need for thinking of all treatment as a combination of techniques individualized for the benefit of a particular patient.

Use of Pharmacological Agents

There are four basic steps in deciding to use pharmacological agents. The first is to assess the patient's experiences and feelings about drugs.

The decision to use a sedative hypnotic is more often a reflection of the dentist's personal style and preference than of the patient's. However, the patient's drug history, personal preferences, and expectations must also be assessed, for if they are not, the probability of successful management is reduced. Some patients strongly believe in the efficacy of drugs. Others fear the effects of the drugs themselves or fear the loss of control inherent in taking a psychoactive substance. For example, some do not want their minds clouded by a mind-altering drug. Conversely, some patients initially insist on a pharmacological solution to their fear. While all patient requests should be taken seriously, initial requests for heavy sedation may reflect a lack of awareness of the options that are available. Thinking that they "can't cope," patients may pin their hopes on a drug that will do the coping for them.

When planning treatment, clinicians should ask the following questions: Does the patient have a preference for or against drugs in general? How safe does the patient perceive the dental environment to be? What is the patient's history with sedative and psychoactive agents, including alcohol?

If the patient thinks that dental treatment is safe, her overall trust is high, and she simply considers herself poor at coping with fear, she is a good candidate for pharmacological therapies. On the other hand, a patient who worries that treatment may not be safe, or exhibits a low level of trust, is a poor candidate. The use of an anti-anxiety agent *decreases* the sense of control.

Secondly, it is important to determine what the drug is being used for. Sedative-hypnotics should be targeted and used for a specific purpose. For patients who have a major problem with anticipation, drugs may aid sleep the night before treatment. For others, a drug may lower the arousal or upset they feel when arriving at the office or initially seated in the dental operatory. Still others may tend to be calm until specific procedures, such as local anesthetic injections, actually begin. The support the patient needs can range from enhanced relaxation to something that will help them avoid experiencing or remembering the actual procedure. Once a drug is chosen, be sure to discuss:

- How will the patient feel now and later?
- What are the potential side effects?
- Can the patient drive a car or take a bus or taxi afterwards?
- Will he need an escort or someone to stay with him?

Third, it is essential to identify in advance what a patient will be doing and thinking during treatment, to communicate that even with a strong drug the patient still has the responsibility to cope. In our experience, patients are sometimes "oversold" on what a given drug, such as nitrous oxide, will do. This can lead to dissatisfaction or the feeling that, "the drug didn't work for me." Thus, patients might be told that a drug is a relaxant and will make them feel more comfortable, but it is a mistake to imply that they will have no worries or feel an absence of sensation. The clinician must communicate to the patient that he cannot simply rely on the effect of the drug alone, and the clinician must consider what else needs to be done to prepare him so that he will behave predictably and appropriately when a drug is administered in association with dental treatment. This is why combining pharmacological and behavioral therapies is so important. Predictability is not only needed to insure efficient treatment, it also essential for patient safety. Control strategies should also be discussed. Should there be a signal the patient can use to stop treatment? Should there be a structured time or provision for rest breaks during an aversive procedure? Such steps enhance positive outcomes because the patient develops the view that they, and not the drug alone, were influential in obtaining a good outcome.

Fourth, in the presence of pharmacological agents, inexperienced dental personnel often act as if the patient were not present, and that the drug will insure that things will go smoothly. In contrast, the truly effective dental provider will coach and encourage patients to use coping skills and play an active behavioral role even when drugs are "on board." For very fearful patients, or those who have no experience with such agents, we recommend a pretreatment, supervised experience with the drug in the office before the actual dental treatment. It allows the practitioner to optimize the dose and the patient to practice coping skills in a brief simulated appointment. This is especially important with nitrous oxide (Weinstein *et al.*, 1988). Extraneous conversation, unrelated to the patient, should be avoided.

What Drug? What Dose?

In surveys where dentists are questioned, wide ranges of drug dosages and approaches are reported. Overall, we strongly recommend that less is better. With less sedation, patients can cope and are more likely to remember the experience and attribute their success to their own efforts. Conversely, when a patient reports that a drug is not having the intended effect or is anxious, negotiation can take place. A more effective dose or a different drug may be appropriate.

Oral Agents

For preoperative insomnia, triazolam (Halcion®, 0.125-0.25 mg for a 75 kg adult) 30 minutes before bed may be helpful. Where triazolam is not available, a similar dose of alprazolam (Xanax®) may be equally effective. If the drug is administered sublingually and allowed to dissolve, peak plasma levels are achieved more rapidly than if it is swallowed (Garzone & Kroboth, 1989). Similarly, this dose of either drug may be helpful if taken 30 to 45 minutes before treatment when the problem is arousal in anticipation of the procedure (Milgrom *et al.*, 1994). The effects of these drugs are subject to diurnal patterns, and afternoon administration may result in more sedation than does morning administration.

For healthy subjects, there is some evidence that carefully individualized doses of the *beta*-adrenergic blocking agent propranolol may help physiologically aroused patients feel more comfortable (Liu *et al.*, 1991). The optimal patient for this drug is one who experiences a high heart rate in the waiting room which accelerates when he is seated in the dental chair. We monitor such patients continuously with an inexpensive hand-held portable heart rate monitor available through exercise and cycle shops. The noninvasive probe for the monitor clips to an ear lobe. Typically the rate is 100 to 120 beats-per-minute. Initially we dispense an oral dose of 80 mg and observe the heart rate for 20 to 30 minutes. The rate should drop 10-20 beats per minute. If it does not drop, we dispense a second similar dose and observe the patient further. With control of breathing, and the second dose, the patient should see her heart rate return nearly to the normal range. This type of *biofeedback* can be extremely helpful to the right patient. *Beta*-blockers do not cause strong sedative effects and should not prevent most patients from driving a car or going back to work. On the other hand, clinicians should always be aware of the patients' physical status and knowledgeable about the contraindications for using this and other drug classes. When in doubt, a medical consultation is appropriate.

The first time you administer the benzodiazepines to any patient in the office, arrangements should be made for his transportation. Many patients can drive or travel on public transport without difficulty, but you should use caution at least the first time. Both triazolam and alprazolam are short acting and patients recover rapidly; diazepam is much more long acting and, in our experience, it is somewhat less predictable. It appears safe to give children adult doses if they are healthy and monitored properly. (Quarnstrom *et al.*, 1992; Berthold *et al.*, 1993).

Elderly patients should always receive 50 percent of the normal dose given to younger patients. Moreover, because chronic and often inappropriate benzodiazepine use is high in this population, it behooves the clinician to be aware of the patient's history and alert for tolerance to benzodiazepines. Monitor the elderly very carefully. Slips and falls in the office or in the home afterwards are significant liability concerns.

Nitrous Oxide

Nitrous oxide is administered at concentrations from 20 percent to 50 percent with oxygen. In practice the doses delivered are much lower than the machine settings, as leakage, mouth breathing, and talking affect the outcome. Teaching patients to breathe the gas in a practice session is particularly effective in titrating to the desired effect. Patients should be told that the effects are general relaxation rather than tingling in the extremities because such specific feelings are highly unpredictable. Nitrous oxide is most helpful in reducing the aversiveness of mildly uncomfortable, fairly short procedures. If the drug is apparently not effective, the reason is usually an ill-prepared patient or an inappropriate procedure rather than too low a dose. A dentist who is constantly increasing the dose will soon abandon the use of nitrous oxide.

Intravenous Sedation

Few general practitioners will employ parenteral medications for sedation because of training, safety, and liability concerns. Nevertheless, some patients will require alternatives to oral sedatives described earlier. Using intravenous combinations of benzodiazepines, narcotics, and barbiturates is especially popular among clinicians in hospital settings. They are often helpful when a patient is having extensive dental procedures, when she travels long distances for care, and where a normal doctor-patient relationship is not required.

It is difficult to interpret much of the outcomes research in this area as patients who volunteer for studies are frequently not typical of community practice patients and are often not very fearful. Nevertheless, there is evidence that IV drug strategies involving combinations of benzodiazepines and other drugs ameliorate intra-operative anxiety (Milgrom *et al.*, 1994).

An Alternative to IV Medications

Nitrous oxide combined with oral triazolam is a safe and effective alternative to parenteral sedation for some patients. In one well done study, 0.25 mg triazolam was combined with 40 percent nitrous oxide with oxygen and found efficacious. No advantage was found for larger doses of triazolam (Kaufman *et al.*, 1993).

SUMMARY

In this chapter we discussed the importance of identifying and teaching the fearful patient a skill he can use during treatment to help him reduce his fear and emotional upset. Coping strategies fall into two broad categories: physical relaxation strategies such as breathing or muscle relaxation, and cognitive strategies such as distraction or mental focusing. Making the patient an active participant in the treatment process enhances his sense of control and self-efficacy. It also lessens their dependence of relying solely on your skills to make the experience tolerable.

Once a patient has identified a strategy to help combat his fear, we recommend utilizing "practice sessions." Graduated exposure and systematic desensitization provide the patient a safe structured environment in which to rehearse newly acquired skills before proceeding with treatment.

Finally, we examined the factors to consider in using a pharmacological adjunct to help reduce a patients's anxiety and then discussed some of the more commonly used drugs in dental practice.

QUESTIONS AND EXERCISES

1. To illustrate the role of anticipation, think back to the last time you experienced some significant anxiety, such as, the last important examination that you took. What bodily responses can you remember? What did you think of before the actual experience? As it turned out, did you need to worry ahead of time? Were you able to talk yourself out of the feelings? If so, what did you tell yourself? If not, what could you have done differently?

2. Describe how you would recommend a friend overcome worrying, anticipatory, thoughts which lead to procrastination or avoidance of a situation.

3. List as many distracters as you can think of that might conceivably be adapted to use in the dental operatory.

4. Describe the role of positive and negative expectations and self-efficacy in overcoming fear.

5. What are the four basic steps you should take before deciding to utilize a pharmacological adjunct?

SEVEN

Pain and
Pain Management

- Conceptualizing Pain
- Fear and Pain
- Coping with Anxiety and Pain
- Controlling Pain
- Enhancing Post-Treatment Comfort

As we discussed in Chapter 2, unpleasant direct and indirect experiences play a major role in the etiology of dental fear. Moreover, pain control is an important clinical requirement in treating fearful patients. Thus, in large part this chapter is intended as a bridge between our general discussion of fear and its psychological and pharmacological management, and specific fear-related management problems.

There are, however, two additional reasons for a special chapter devoted to this subject. First, although pain control is not a new subject for the dentist, we have found that many inaccuracies and errors occur in this area, suggesting that dentists are failing to adopt

HERMAN®

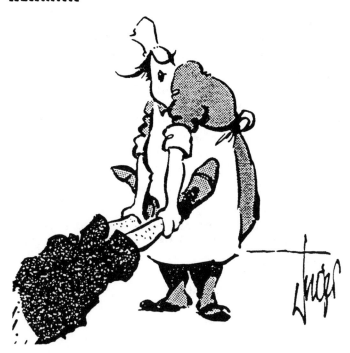

"Mr. White is here for his annual checkup, doctor."

new information. Second, many dental personnel see anxiety control, especially through the modalities of nitrous oxide, oral premedication, and IV sedation, as the *primary* means of treating the fearful patient. We hope to describe what we have found to be the appropriate uses of these drugs while also strongly suggesting complementary behavioral strategies.

CONCEPTUALIZING PAIN

The first section of this chapter defines what we mean by pain, specifies two theories of pain and their clinical implications, and establishes the relationship between anxiety and pain.

This chapter also examines cultural and personality factors related to pain. We next discuss in-operatory pain control and focus on topical and injectable anesthetics and the post-operative management of pain. Other drugs used in the operatory, such as nitrous oxide, are discussed in Chapter 6.

If pain is not just a sensation, what is it? That question cannot be answered simply because pain is a complex phenomenon. Sternbach (1968) described pain as an abstract concept that refers to (1) a personal, private sensation of hurt; (2) a harmful stimulus that signals current or impending tissue damage; and (3) a pattern of responses that operates to protect the organism from harm. In some respects, pain is a sensation and in other respects it is a psychological phenomenon that allows us to escape or avoid trauma.

Consider the definition of pain arrived at by an international group of experts and published by *Pain* in 1979 IASP Subcommittee on Taxonomy.

> ... An unpleasant sensory and emotional experience associated with actual or potential tissue damage or described in terms of damage.
> ... Pain is always subjective. Each individual learns the application of the word with experiences related to injury in early life. Biologists recognize that those stimuli which cause pain are liable to damage tissue. Accordingly, pain is that experience which we associate with actual or potential tissue damage. It is unquestionably a sensation in a part or parts of the body but is also always unpleasant and therefore also an emotional experience. Experiences which resemble pain, e.g.,

pricking, but are not unpleasant, should not be called pain.

Many people report pain in the absence of tissue damage or any likely pathophysiological cause; usually this happens for psychological reasons. There is no way to distinguish their experience from that due to tissue damage if we take the subjective report. *If they regard their experience as pain and if they report it in the same ways as pain caused by tissue damage, it should be accepted as pain.* [Our Italics] This definition avoids tying pain to the stimulus. Activity induced in the nociceptor and nociceptive pathways by a noxious stimulus is not pain, which is always a psychological state, even though we may well appreciate that pain most often has a proximate physical cause.

These descriptions and definitions make it clear that the pain is not merely a response to an external stimulus. Rather, it is clearly a subjective psychological state, and as such, is influenced by much more than the associated physical stimulus.

Two contrasting examples may be helpful as we think about the wide range of pain responses presented clinically by dental patients.

The first is Karen, a 22-year-old student, who is caries-free but has localized gingivitis because of poor hygiene in some areas of her mouth. She reports the sensation of the rubber prophylaxis cup on her teeth as unbearable pain. In such a patient, diagnostic procedures that rely on patient self-report, such as vitality testing, are especially problematic (Eli, 1993).

The second example is Richard, a 35-year-old construction worker, who often experiences bruises and other minor injuries at work. He was seen for a periodontal abscess. He had avoided treatment because he thought the swelling might be cancer. The area was anesthetized and debrided. Repeatedly during the procedure he tensed up the muscles of his face and brought his hands up as if in pain. However, when questioned he said he was only anticipating it hurting.

Theories of Pain

There have been many theories of pain. Van Frey in 1894 (Melzack & Wall, 1965) presented an extremely influential *specificity* theory.

Specific pain receptors, when stimulated, were believed to result in pain. He hypothesized a one-to-one relationship between stimulation of nerve endings and the sensation of pain. Although there were alternative theories which postulated that impulses were coded or patterned at the periphery and then modulated during transmission by central nervous system inputs, the specificity theory had the most adherents. Medical and dental texts considered pain in those terms. Detailed reviews of pain can be found in Clark and Hunt (1971), Melzack (1968), and Melzack and Wall (1965).

In the last three decades, there has been evidence that specificity theory is insufficient to account for the phenomenon of clinical pain. Hill and associates (1952) showed that reduction of experimentally induced anxiety in subjects in laboratory experiments resulted in lowered intensity of pain. They have also shown that morphine reduces pain if the anxiety level is high, but has no effect if anxiety is low.

Similarly, Beecher (1959) has argued that it is not possible to equate laboratory pain with clinical pain. Although morphine can be extremely effective in reducing pain reactions in clinical situations, it cannot be distinguished from saline in diminishing laboratory pain. In the clinic, placebo pain medications are effective in about one-third of the uses, but in the laboratory this percentage is reduced to almost zero. The missing ingredients in the laboratory are the anxiety and upset of the patient. *Reducing pain in the clinic often involves reducing anxiety.*

Beecher's classical (1959) study of soldiers also illustrates this point. Of 215 men who were seriously wounded in a battle, only 25 percent wanted a narcotic for relief. In comparison, over 80 percent of civilians with a similar surgical wound made under anesthesia requested narcotics. Beecher interpreted the difference in responses to the significance each group attributed to the wounds. In wartime, a battle wound meant relief to a soldier, return to home, perhaps as a hero. In civilian life the surgery means disruption, cost, and disability. The setting influences the reaction to painful stimuli. Theorizing about pain must include such emotional and motivational factors.

One more bit of evidence: surgeons have attempted to use the knowledge gained in the laboratory to alleviate clinical pain by surgically severing branches of major facial nerves. This work, for example with atypical facial pain, produces unreliable results. Thus, the evidence for the success of cutting the nerve between the peripheral damage and the CNS gives little support for the specificity approach.

Laboratory study has focused on the sensory nature of pain. Pain receptors have been mapped, and neural pathways from peripheral to central areas have been established. However, many such studies have excluded from investigation the psychological component of pain. Szasz (1957) theorized that laboratory studies have no relevance for clinical practice. The subjects know that the pain will end soon and that no permanent tissue damage will occur. He concludes that the laboratory is not a useful place to examine pain responsivity, since it is impossible to arouse substantial anxiety in that setting. Dworkin and Chen (1982), 25 years later, provided the first real experimental evidence that laboratory investigations may minimize pain responses. These researchers found that a clinical pain-producing dental situation yielded heightened pain and increased sensitivity compared with the pain experienced in a research laboratory using identical stimulation. We cannot overlook the capacity of psychological variables, such as patient appraisal of threat, to lower pain thresholds. Findings from laboratory studies of anesthesia and pain that do not elicit anxiety may not generalize very well to clinical practice.

The Gate Control Theory (Melzack & Wall, 1965) has been the most influential and important contemporary theory of pain perception. In short, the theory proposes that transmission of a noxious stimulus through a dorsal spinal gating mechanism is contingent not only on the arrival of the stimulus, but also on other events in the periphery and on the set of the brain, which determines whether to permit the message to arrive. The authors suggested that three psychological processes contribute to a person's perception of pain: the discrimination of sensory input, the subjective reaction to such input, and the cognitive evaluation of sensation. More than any other theoretical approach, Gate Control Theory emphasizes the large role of psychological variables and how they affect the reaction to pain.

The Gate Control Theory has been criticized because it does not account fully for all the neurophysiological data available today. We refer readers who are interested in greater detail to Melzack and Wall (1965, 1970) and Melzack (1973).

Fordyce (1976), Sternbach and Fordyce (1975), and Gentry and Bernal (1977) have proposed that such behavior, as moaning, crying, distorted gait, or taking medication for pain relief, are important components of pain. These researchers theorize that much of pain involves overt action and modification of this behavior is important in pain control.

FEAR AND PAIN

Before discussing the relationship of pain to fear, it is necessary to describe the theory of emotion and the importance of anticipation. The relationship between fear and pain is not simple. Some research shows that initially, fear inhibits pain, and that this inhibition occurs on the perceptual side, via descending pathways to interneurons in the dorsal horn of the spinal cord. This gating, mediated by endorphins and enkephalins, occurs at the first afferent synapse.

Endorphins and Pain Behavior

The research on opiate-like substances in brain tissue has promise of explaining the relationship between psychological and physiological functioning. Morphine-like agents, endorphins ("endorphin" is a contraction of "endogenous" and "morphine"), have been identified and are subjects of wide-ranging research—from biochemical to behavioral. Stressors, especially fear, are believed to trigger the release of endorphins from the pituitary, resulting in an analgesic effect. As the stressor continues, naloxone, which antagonizes the analgesic, is released and pain is enhanced.

This is often the situation we face clinically. Those who are fearful in shorter restorative appointments do not show much upset; however, longer appointments are usually traumatic. Once a patient's fears are allayed, moreover, pain is less likely to occur. Another indication that fear promotes pain is the widespread use of sedative-hypnotics and alcohol to treat and prevent pain. Many patients perceive that 5–10 mg of diazepam or an ounce of alcohol are useful before dental treatment.

The principle is clear: *deal with the fear first*, and then pain will be a minor problem. But why should this occur? Fear is said to activate the endorphins; it should reduce pain induced by noxious stimuli.

How can it sensitize the pain system? Bolles and Faneslow (1980), in their model of fear and pain, suggest that muscle tension may be a factor. Anxiety produces muscle tension. This tension has a variety of physical effects including pain. Another complementary explanation is that it is not pain that causes the suffering reported by patients, but fear itself. The agony of a traumatic dental appointment may be due more to the fear than the pain. Patients may report the experience as painful because they can identify a fearful stimulus. The distress is not caused by the stimulus, i.e., the drilling activated pain. Rather, it is caused by mislabeling the distress, such as being confined in a frightening situation. The mislabeling is hypothesized to arise from the fact that the patient's attention is focused, because of expectation, on the fearful stimulus. We have all learned that such a predicament—the inability to fight or flee—is painful. However, the dominant motivational system is fear, not pain.

Psychologists have presented other theories about the relationship between pain and fear. As we discussed in Chapter 2, the theories emphasize the conditioning of fear to stimuli a patient senses or thinks of as painful. Clinically and experimentally, it is well established that when patients are anxious, they have a "lower pain threshold." In fact, all autonomic activation, not only fear, causes lower thresholds for pain and lower pain tolerance. Anticipation before the dental treatment itself has an effect upon pain threshold and tolerance. Patients who experience prolonged anticipatory arousal, usually with some form of thoughts about catastrophe, are often not able to control themselves during the dental appointment. This arousal usually makes itself felt hours or even days before the appointment and elicits additional fear. Now the patient fears not only dental treatment, but also the aversiveness of his own arousal and its accompanying thoughts. Such situations often result in the patient being overwhelmed. His perceived lack of control—an inability to respond with desired fight or flight—also contributes to the problem. This patient becomes panicky and looks physically drained. He may flee the dental chair in tears before treatment, avert the head during injection, or bite the dentist's finger. He may report nausea, shortness of breath, or dizziness. He may perspire profusely. This process is outlined in the model below.

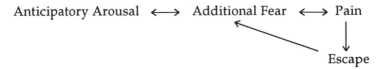

Note the arrows that go in both directions: arousal causes additional fear, and additional fear enhances future fear and arousal. Pain leads not only to escape, but also to additional future fear and arousal. Effective patient management focuses both on in-chair anxiety and on the anticipatory arousal and its labeling.

Cultural Factors and Pain

Differences in how people from different cultures react to pain have received considerable study, and it is apparent that cultural training greatly influences these differences. In 1952, Zbrowski's classic work, *People in Pain*, highlighted different perceptions and responses to pain. For instance, Jewish and Italian patients responded more emotionally than others to pain and tended to magnify it; "Old Americans" were more stoic than others; Irish patients tended to deny pain. Since then, many scholarly papers have been presented on this subject. African-Americans, Eskimos, American Indians, Puerto Ricans, and other ethnic and racial groups have been studied. Weisenberg (1977a) reviewed these studies and placed them in a theoretical framework.

According to Weisenberg, major differences between cultural groups seem to be related to pain tolerance (the extent of noxious stimuli) rather than to the threshold discrimination of pain (initial level reported as pain) as a sensation. Underlying attitude differences and reactions to anxiety appear to be a major source of these differences in pain tolerance. Weisenberg comments:

> When outside sensory means for evaluation are reduced, the individual turns toward his social environment for validation of his judgments. Since pain is a private, ambiguous situation, comparison with others helps to determine what reactions are appropriate. Is it permissible to cry? Does one have to grin and bear it? When is it permissible to ask for help?

People learn many of their anxieties and reactions by observing others. This process takes place in childhood, within families, as well as in social settings. For example, Craig and Best (1977) have shown that pain tolerance is subject to the social influence of models in a laboratory setting. Shoben and Borland (1954) have shown that experiences and attitudes of family members are very important in determining a person's reaction to dental treatment. Similarly, Johnson and Baldwin (1968) found that children whose mothers had high anxiety scores showed more anxious behavior than children of mothers with low anxiety.

We need to raise a few more points about the influence of cultural factors and pain. Some findings ("myths" as Zbrowski called them in 1952) are based on very few observations in situations where the subjects' reactions may have been biased by the testing situation itself. For example, initial research by white researchers on pain tolerance of African-Americans predicted low pain tolerance (Katz, 1964). However, more recent studies report no difference between black and white obstetrical patients (Weisenberg, 1977b) and medical students (Merskey & Spear, 1964). More importantly, these generalizations are often not predictive of the individual patient in the dental setting.

COPING WITH ANXIETY AND PAIN

Fearful people often act as if their behaviors are uncontrollable. Thus, we begin by telling patients in the Dental Fears Research Clinic how their attitudes, feeling, and attention can actually alter their tolerance to pain. We explain how the tension from inappropriate fight-flight responses increases their sensitivity to pain. The arousal *itself* is aversive (Bolles & Fanselow, 1980). Thus, patients often contribute to their own discomfort: when they are upset they are actually more likely to feel pain—real physical pain (Sternbach, 1968). Therefore, we explain that their job is to control their own emotions while our job is to assist them and to make the actual sensations as minimal as possible.

To demonstrate this principle clinically have a patient clench one hand while leaving the other relaxed. Pinch both hands between the thumb and first finger. The results will be that the "relaxed" hand feels less pain.

Knowing how the patient ordinarily copes with stressful events may be important as you develop an optimal dental pain control strategy. A few dimensions have been identified as important and can be readily assessed.

Can the patient respond to stressors in his life with some sort of conscious coping *strategy*, or does the patient respond only with *catastrophizing* thoughts? Chaves and Brown (1978) interviewed a series of patients undergoing dental treatment. From this interview, they classified patients according to whether or not they used a coping strategy to reduce stress, and if not, whether they had catastrophizing thoughts. They found that patients used cognitive coping strategy experienced less stress than patients whose cognitive activity was characterized as catastrophizing. Similarly, in 1974, Chaves and Barber reported in an experimental study that the greater the amount of time subjects used either the researchers' cognitive strategy or their own strategy, the greater the pain reduction.

In our experience, some intensely fearful patients do not feel that they have the ability to generate a pain coping strategy. This may not be necessary. Chaves and Brown (1974) found that it may be more important to avoid catastrophizing than to engage in positive coping. Clinically, identification and elimination of catastrophic ideation is always our first priority. Catastrophizing is much worse than not being able to generate a strategy.

In both the Chaves and Brown work and the more recent study of Richardson and Kleinknecht (1984), catastrophizers rated their dental procedures as more stressful than did copers. Clearly, as noted earlier in this chapter, the stressfulness and pain of the dental experience are magnified by those who tend to show catastrophizing ideation.

Examples of Coping Strategies

Jack: Just like placid thoughts, pictures ... I let my mind wander. Just think on different things like 1 look around and observe things in the room and let them bring my attention to them rather than what's going on in my mouth.

Jennifer: Well, I just tried basically in a philosophic way not to identify with the body. ... Basically I was thinking of a mantra while it was taking place. To just negate is not enough—you have to have something to engage the mind also. So I was trying to get the mind not to think about what was going on in the body.

Martin: I just try and prepare myself. You know it's going to hurt so I tell myself: "Just be ready for it—think about something else." And I tense up more or less when he puts it in and then I just relax and that's about it.

(Adapted from Chaves & Brown, 1974)

The Influence of Personality

Many personality traits of normal people have been associated with reactions to pain. A review of the literature yields conflicting results. Further, the different definitions of personality make comparisons between studies hazardous. Moreover, most studies evaluate long-term chronic pain and its determinants. Acute pain, whether pathologic (e.g., toothache or abscess) or iatrogenic (e.g., injection or drilling) is the kind of pain we refer to when we think of going to the dentist. Reactions to acute and chronic pain are different (Sternbach, 1968; Fordyce, 1976).

Sensitizers versus Repressors. This dimension of personality focuses on styles of handling information. Does the patient try to cope by actively trying to deal with the stressor or does he try to reduce input? People who welcome information, enjoy explanations of diagnostic and treatment procedures, and want to view the treatment may be labeled as monitors or "sensitizers." Those who avoid information and are upset by knowing what is going on may be labeled "repressors" or blunters. They show different patterns of pre- and post-operative anxiety and respond differently to information, as you would predict. Pain responses also seem to be different (Neufeld & Davidson, 1971). Knowledge of where the patient lies on the sensitization-repression (monitor-blunter) continuum will help you develop a successful strategy. Would information and explanation be very useful for a repressor? Or would a sensitizer like to listen to music? Hardly.

Locus of Control. This dimension of personality, which focuses on beliefs, has been widely studied. Briefly, locus of control is a concept regarding the degree to which people see themselves as being in control and responsible for what happens to them. A person with an "external" locus of control believes that whatever happens to him is a result of luck, fate, chance, of powerful others. For example, if he fails a test, it is because the test was unfair, the teacher inadequate. The person with an "internal" locus of control believes that he is in control of what happens. If he fails a test, he believes that it was because he did not study enough.

There is evidence that the scales that measure this personality dimension are useful predispositional measures. For example, Seeman and Evans (1962) found that patients with internal locus of control were better informed about their disease and asked more questions than did others. Johnson and colleagues (1971) found that surgical patients with internal locus of control received more doses of analgesics than did those exhibiting external locus of control. None of the dosages were extreme, and taking the analgesic can be interpreted as coping or adaptive behavior. In fact, it appears that patients with external locus of control requested insufficient medication to control post-operative discomfort. Neverlien (1988) found external locus of control was related to anxiety scores. Houston (1972) found that subjects with internal locus of control performed better on a task when told ahead of time that they could avoid shock contingent on their performance, whereas those with external locus of control performed better when told that they could not avoid shock. Similarly, Auerbach and colleagues (1976), found that in a group of people with internal locus of control, those who viewed videotapes providing specific information about an imminent tooth extraction showed better adjustment during surgery than those who saw a general information tape about the clinic. Conversely, subjects with external locus of control responded more favorably to the general information tape. A number of medical and dental studies, such as that by Duke and Cohen (1974), indicate that people with internal locus of control respond better to preventive and other recommendations that require active patient involvement; those with an external locus of control are believed to require more guidance and structuring. Examples from the 1966 version of the Internal-External (I-E) scale, developed by Julian Rotter, are presented below. Patients are instructed to choose either "a" or "b" for each item.

---

1. a. Children get into trouble because their parents punish them too much.

    b. The trouble with most children nowadays is that their parents are too easy with them.

2. a. Many of the unhappy things in people's lives are partly due to bad luck.

    b. People's misfortunes result from the mistakes they make.

This scale can be used clinically to better understand a patient who can't describe clearly how much responsibility he will take for his own care. For example, will the patient practice relaxation exercises at home? Or follow oral self-care instructions?

Though belief in the efficacy of one's actions is an important personality dimension to be assessed, other aspects of control, independent of personality, are also important. Many patients who generally are in control of their lives feel vulnerable and unable to control the perceived danger of a dental appointment. Most of us prefer to have at least some control over an aversive event, and there is evidence that control over the pain situation can reduce stress and pain reactions. More about the issue of control may be found in Chapter 5.

Suggestibility. Research that seeks personality correlates of both waking and hypnotic suggestibility have not been very successful, although there are some useful results. Children between the ages of 7 and 14 have been found to be significantly more suggestible than adults (Barber & Calverley, 1963), possibly because children are usually quite dependent on others. Consequently, it may be easier to establish rapport, and then trust, with them than with adults. Some investigators have found significant correlations between dependency and suggestibility. Similarly, there is recent evidence that people who are more trusting are more suggestible (Periera & Austrin, 1980). Further, a silent, passive demeanor has been found to be helpful (Reyher et al., 1970). Suggestible subjects are less vigilant, restrict attention in peripheral visual fields, and are less responsive to auditory stimuli (Smyth, 1981).

Researchers have found that suggestibility is primarily determined by situations. That is, it is strongly influenced by the patient's expectations and his relationship with the clinician. Thus, the clinician's personal characteristics may be important because the patient's confidence in the clinician is important. Though prestige and technical competence may contribute to patient suggestibility, there is evidence that the status of the title of "doctor" or "dentist" may not be sufficient. Warmth may be more important (Smyth, 1981). Gryll and Katahn (1978) found that patients' feelings of pain from an injection were influenced by the clinician's personal warmth and by the patients' confidence that the dentist could control pain.

CONTROLLING PAIN

Topical and Local Anesthetics

Anesthetic drugs are very important in pain control, a key modality in ensuring a pain-free and relatively comfortable experience for the fearful patient. Surprisingly, few clinicians completely understand the effect of these potent drugs.

In this section, we will review the basic mechanism and characteristics of topical and local anesthetics and then discuss two clinical problems encountered with fearful patients: anesthetic failure and adverse effects. It is beyond the scope of this text to teach local anesthetic technique. We refer readers to Malamed, *Handbook of Local Anesthesia* (1990), and similar texts for more complete information.

A good source of information on anesthetic drugs used in dentistry is Neidle and Yagiela, *Pharmacology and Therapeutics for Dentistry* (1989). The mainstay of anesthetics used for topical application in dentistry is benzocaine (Americaine®, Hurricaine®). Benzocaine preparations are sold as 20% gels, ointment, pastes, and solutions. A similar but potentially more toxic gel is tetracaine (Cetacaine®) which is 2% tetracaine, 14% benzocaine, and 2% butyl aminobenzoate. Because of the vehicles used to carry these anesthetics, they tend to remain at the site of action. These agents may also be available as a spray. But you must use extreme caution with these sprays, because it is very difficult to control the dosing and there is potential for overdose. Only devices with metered delivery should be used.

The dental hygienists in the Dental Fears Research Clinic favor dyclonine hydrochloride, which is sold as a 0.5% and 1% solution (Dyclone®). Before scaling and root planing, they place the solutions in the gingival sulcus with a cotton pledget, and then wait 2–3 minutes for the solution to work. Dyclonine hydrochloride may be useful for patients who are allergic benzocaine. They also employ 0.717% stannous fluoride (Dentin Bloc™) topically to reduce dentinal hypersensitivity before scaling and root planing. The following example is a typical case.

> Val, a 47-year old nurse, grew up in a rural area where dental care was described as brutal. Whenever she had her teeth cleaned it hurt so she avoided the dental hygienist, only making things worse. Luckily, her problem is primarily gingivitis associated with considerable supragingival calculus. Our findings suggest that the dental hygienist never offered any form of pain control during the prophylaxis. After teaching Val some simple relaxation exercises, our senior dental hygienist used topical anesthetic to reduce the discomfort. For this initial experience, she also divided the treatment into two shorter visits. Val described the cleaning as the best she ever had.

The newest approach to topical anesthetic is EMLA cream, a mixture of 2.5% lidocaine and 2.5% prilocaine (Astra®). This agent contains no preservative and can be used with patients who are allergic to *p*-aminobenzoic acid. Until recently, it was used primarily for dermal applications, particularly as a topical anesthetic before intravenous line placement with children. Svensson and Petersen (1992) have recently suggested that EMLA cream, covered with a carboxymethylcellulose oral bandage (Orahesive Oral Bandage®) for five minutes, is better than placebo in preventing pain during experimental injections involving the greater palatine and incisive foramens. Similar responses have been shown in response to stimulation from an argon laser (Svensson *et al.*, 1993).

Injectable local anesthetics were introduced early in the 20th century. Procaine (Novocaine®) was the first practical drug and although it was thought likely to produce allergic responses, it remained in use until the late 1940s. Lidocaine (Xylocaine®, Octocaine®, Alphacaine®), introduced in 1948, has become the most commonly used dental anesthetic drug. It produces more dependable pulpal and soft tissue anesthesia than procaine and has low allergic potential.

Other drugs, such as mepivacaine and prilocaine, were introduced later and have been reported to have longer duration without vasoconstrictors. Otherwise, their mechanism of action is similar to that of lidocaine.

The newer drugs are classified as amides because of their chemical structure. Procaine is an ester-type anesthetic. The anesthetics work by crossing neuronal membranes and acting on the inner surface of the axonal membrane, blocking both generation and conduction of nerve impulses.

Drug Formulations

In the United States, dental anesthetics are primarily sold in 1.8-ml glass carpules (2.2 ml in Great Britain) containing anesthetic agent, sulfite preservative,* and a vasoconstrictor. Nearly all the drugs used in dentistry today are of the amide class. The key distinction between the drugs is length of action, with the most common drugs (lidocaine, mepivacaine) being relatively medium acting, and less common drugs (e.g., bupivacaine, etidocaine) being long acting. The duration depends on the drug itself, the vasoconstrictor, and site of injection. While not widely understood, the duration of pulpal anesthesia of all the agents containing vasoconstrictor, even the long-acting drugs, is roughly the same. The longer action is limited to soft tissue analgesia. Table 7-1 lists the drugs commonly used in dentistry.

TABLE 7-1
Amide Local Anesthetic Drugs

Chemical Name	Representative Brand Names	Relative Duration
Lidocaine	Xylocaine®	Medium
Mepivacaine	Carbocaine®	Medium
Prilocaine	Citanest®	Medium
Bupivacaine	Marcaine®	Long

Since 1981 manufacturers have begun removing paraben from local anesthetics because it may cause hypersensitivity. However, some drug formulations, especially those sold in Canada, may still contain it.

Dosage. It is not known exactly how much is generally given in dental practice, although it is likely that one or two 1.8-ml cartridges of medium-duration drugs are routinely given. These dosages are far below the maximum safe dosage levels and may account for many reports of inadequate anesthesia.

The maximum adult dosages for local anesthetic drugs (Neidle & Yagiela, 1989) to be used in dental therapy are given in Table 7-2. Dosing for children should be done on a mg/kg basis.

Onset. Many of the fear reactions we have seen in patients referred to our clinic have been labeled by dentists as reactions to an anesthetic drug or vasoconstrictor. A good part of the problem may be the long period many practitioners wait between injections, testing for anesthesia, and beginning actual operations. This is particularly true in the mandible, where it is not uncommon for 15–20 minutes to elapse between the first injection of a single cartridge and then another, often with the message from the dentist that the first "did not work." As suggested above, one cartridge may provide inadequate anesthesia for operative dentistry in some areas of the mouth.

However, a major misconception is that anesthesia onset is very slow and that waiting 10-15 minutes helps. Since problems occur most often in the inferior alveolar block injection, this is a good example of this faulty perception. Research shows that 90 percent of patients will have the onset of lip symptoms in 65–75 seconds, with onset of long-acting drugs taking somewhat longer than onset in medium-acting drugs. Periosteal anesthesia was obtained in over 90 percent of cases in about three minutes.

We will discuss injection technique in more detail later this chapter; however, our clinical practice is to give a single cartridge, wait about one minute for the onset of soft tissue symptoms, and proceed "painlessly" to administer a full dose of the drug. This avoids the "aura" of anesthetic failure and the inevitable increase in patient anxiety associated with the anticipation that "I might get hurt." Once patients realize that follow-up injections do not hurt, most relax.

TABLE 7-2
Maximum Adult Dosages for Local Anesthetic Drugs

Drug	Maximum Dose
Prilocaine	600 mg
Lidocaine	500 mg
Mepivacaine	400 mg
Bupivacaine	225 mg

Area of Anesthesia. Some routinely fail to anesthetize a sufficient area to work painlessly. This is particularly true for the palate, where the dentist may perceive injections to be painful. The dentist's reluctance is picked up by the patient and often translated into requests to avoid these injections. Inevitably, however, this results in discomfort during the operative or periodontal procedure. The clinician can use topical anesthesia plus pressure with the butt end of the dental mirror handle or cotton tip applicator to reduce discomfort during injections in the palatal tissue.

Problem of Inadequate Local Anesthesia

Although pain control is considered a requisite of restorative dentistry, and local anesthesia is the method of choice for most patients in the United States and Canada, there are few studies of its success. Textbooks recommend a variety of clinical techniques without consistency in their discussions of success rates. Clinical "failures" are reported to result from very short duration of anesthesia, injection technique, the properties of the anesthetic agent, unusual nerve anatomy, or infection. Malamed, in the *Handbook of Local Anesthesia*, reports successful mandibular block in 80–97 percent of injections, depending on the technique used. He believes that failures are attributable to the density of the mandible, limited accessibility of the nerves, and anatomical variation. He reports a success rate of 95 percent in maxillary injections, which he attributes to less dense bone and easy accessibility, but he does not hypothesize a reason for failures. Similar findings have been reported for failures in local anesthesia for children (Kuster & Rakes, 1987). The usual criterion for anesthesia is sufficient numbness to allow tooth preparation without pain (pulpal anesthesia).

There are two basic types of studies: (1) reports of clinical ob-servations and (2) laboratory studies. Clinical studies often report the incidence of anesthetic failures and identify their cause. Labora-tory studies, in both animals and humans, most often evaluate the dosage-duration relationship for anesthetics and do not address anesthetic failures.

These studies are reviewed in detail by Kaufman, Weinstein, and Milgrom (1984). Although there are many dental and non-dental reports about the relationship between fear and pain, the literature is generally silent on psychological factors that may influence inadequate anesthesia. Factors such as fear are clearly capable of influencing patient response to painful or other stimuli applied after administration of local anesthetic. Thus, these factors may contribute to inadequate anesthesia. Moreover, the relationship between these variables may be reciprocal: fear can lead to inadequate anesthesia and being treated with inadequate anesthesia can increase fear. A recent case provides a good example.

> Susan, a 35-year-old school teacher, was referred to us, in part, because she could not become numb enough to tolerate a crown preparation on tooth number 31. Our findings suggest that the dentist used too little anesthetic and waited too long for anesthesia onset. He also inappropriately with-drew the vasoconstrictor when she complained about her heart racing and being sensitive to the "Novicain." After Susan learned some basic breathing and muscle relaxation skills, which helped to keep her heart rate down, we were able to anesthetize her tooth successfully and complete the crown preparation.

To begin to evaluate the extent of problems with local anesthetics in clinical practice, we randomly selected 200 Washington State general dentists from the Washington State Dental Association directory and surveyed them. Dentists reported giving inadequate anesthesia, on average, for 13 percent of all patients in the previous five days. The vast majority of dentists reported some inadequate anesthesia. Years of practice experience did not influence the rate; practical experience itself did not lead to more successful pain con-trol.

Rates for inadequate anesthesia differed by type of injection.

Mandibular blocks presented the greatest problem, followed by maxillary posterior and maxillary anterior injections. In response to initial anesthetic failure, almost all dentists gave an additional injection. However, disrupted or lengthened patient visits were extremely common. Dentists also indicated that high percentages (47 percent) of patients were fearful or anxious.

If the dentist changes drugs during a treatment visit after failing to achieve anesthesia the first time it may lead to problems of misattribution and problems of adverse effects. See Chapter 8. Giving an anesthetic without a vasoconstrictor may assure inadequate anesthesia and increase the chances of adverse effects, especially if the dentist attempts work with resulting pain (Milgrom *et al.*, 1984). Bernstein and colleagues (1979) have shown that the most highly feared aspects of dentistry are painful dental procedures.

Improving Anesthesia:
attention to patient anxiety and technique

Patient Anxiety. You can take steps to reduce failures and enhance anesthesia. First, you should prepare patients for the injection. Research has shown that relaxed patients achieve greater pain control than those who are tense (Bobey & Davidson, 1970). We recommend that the dental staff observe the patient carefully before starting treatment. Are his respiration and heart rate slow and rhythmic? Or is his breathing quickened and his pulse racing? Are his facial muscles relaxed or tense? Are his hands clenched?. Most patients are able to relax sufficiently by taking a few long breaths, concentrating on exhalation. You might accompany this breathing exercise by the suggestion that it will lead to relaxation and greater comfort during dental procedures. Trust and rapport are essential if this procedure is to be effective. For extremely tense patients, relaxation procedures, hypnosis, or biofeedback in conjunction with relaxation, are effective. Dentists who employ nitrous oxide will find that these approaches can be used both before and during inhalation sedation and will enhance the result. This is also true for dentists who use premedication or IV medications.

Technique. Second, it's a good idea to review and perfect your techniques of administering local anesthesia. This includes the use of topical and injectable anesthetics, and specific communication strategies. Use the topical anesthesic to give the patient the feeling of numbness. Some clinicians do not feel it necessary for pain control but they are losing opportunities for good communication. Often, we find it helpful to place the topical first on the tongue to teach the patient the sensation. Then when it is placed on the gingiva, she will be better able to feel its effect. Often it is helpful to ask the patient to affirm feeling the anesthetic effect of the topical before proceeding with the injection. Because the drug is poorly absorbed it takes 60–90 seconds to have full effect.

Then, inject the local anesthetic slowly to minimize discomfort. During the injection it is helpful to suggest to the patient that she will feel the sensation of numbness spreading and becoming more complete. Use adequate volumes of anesthetic and if the full-blown onset of anesthesia is not forthcoming in two to three minutes, administer an additional volume. Prolonging this time interval is inefficient and does not contribute to a better result. Patients with anesthetic failure histories should be given larger doses initially (Fiset *et al.*, 1989). A form of cross tolerance has been suggested between "street drugs" and alcohol and local anesthetics. Patients with substance abuse histories present potential pain control problems.

Finally, drilling is the only true test of dental anesthesia we have, and some small number of patients will report pain during drilling even when they are relaxed. Painless drilling is one of the miracles of modern dentistry, and under most circumstances, treatment should not proceed if the patient is reporting discomfort. Most often these partially numb patients have subjective signs of soft tissue anesthesia. However, this does not necessarily indicate the presence of pulpal anesthesia. Our experience with patients who have long histories of anesthetic failure is that if we use appropriate relaxation procedures, then supplementary injections (such as the intraseptal or intraligamentary) are effective. However, it is important for the dentist to remain especially objective at this stage. If anesthesia remains inadequate, then perhaps infection or some other biological or anatomical cause is at work.

Using the Vitalometer. Large and small nerve fibers have different sensitivities to the effects of local anesthetics. Larger fibers are more resistant to anesthetic blocking. Thus, it is not unusual for patients to have many of the symptoms of analgesia without being profoundly numb. We often use a pulp vitality tester at this stage with patients for whom poor anesthesia has been a problem. For example, we first establish that the patient can provide reliable feedback on a pretest. Then, after administering a normal dose of anesthetic, we retest the tooth. If we are able to go to the end of the scale we proceed with drilling. Often, however, the patient will respond three-quarters of the way up the tester scale. At that point, an intraligamentary or intraseptal injection and retesting may be necessary. When patients are retested and are able to see the difference in their responses, drilling usually proceeds uneventfully. Our experience has been that drilling will be painful unless the patient is completely insensitive to the pulp tester stimulus.

In situations where repeated injections result in failure, place a sedative filling. We find that patients are able to accept biological explanations for anesthetic failure and are relieved to know that the dentist does not think they are "crazy." Before the next appointment, review the pain control procedures to be used. For generalized anxiety patients we find that an oral premedication or giving the patient additional relaxation exercises to practice at home helps to reduce the anxiety associated with the anesthetic injection. Also, carefully consider collateral nerve supply and give supplementary injections initially. Let the patient know and expect that a stronger, more effective drug or technique is being used now. However, in those situations where the patient is fearful of an adverse reaction to the anesthetic, we would never suggest switching anesthetics unless allergy testing indicated a true reaction. In our experience, under these circumstances anesthesia will be effective, the dentist's reputation will be enhanced, and the patient's comfort increased.

The following case history illustrates how the above principles can be applied.

John, a 30-year-old construction worker, came to our clinic after avoiding dental care for the past 13 years. He reported that as an adult he had difficulty getting numb. "Novocain doesn't work on me. The last time I was injected 11 times with the needle." He reported additional instances of multiple injections without the desired effect. "The pain was always unbearable; the injections don't do their job for me."

We gave John relaxation instructions and he practiced

deep breathing in the chair before treatment. During the initial interview we had learned that he was an avid fisherman. We used this information in guided imaging, and John relaxed. After we applied the topical anesthetic, we injected two cartridges of anesthetic (2% lidocaine with 1:100,000 epinephrine) to anesthetize the upper right first premolar. The decay was deep and John reported minor sensitivity in the pulpal wall area while the decay was being removed. Instead of reinjecting, which might not have been successful and would have reinforced John's expectation that he could not be numb, we placed a sedative filling. The next week the restoration was completed. John reported no discomfort at any of five subsequent restorative appointments. Moreover, at the last appointment, he fell asleep in the chair! Pushing ahead to finish the restoration at the initial appointment might have resulted in a clinical failure.

ENHANCING POST—TREATMENT COMFORT

Dental treatment and the recovery interval are often periods of physical and psychological stress for patients. The physical stress comes from actual tissue damage. The psychological stress can occur because of the patient's expectations of being harmed during treatment, or of experiencing complications following it. It is clear that the degree of physical trauma affects post-operative recovery. However, it has only recently been recognized that psychological factors influence actual physical aspects of post-surgical recovery.

Research by George and colleagues (1980) shows a correlation between healing rate after surgery, the patient's acceptance of his condition, and the *meaning* of the event to the patient. Patients who attached a positive meaning to their situation healed more quickly, perceived their problems as surmountable, and saw their condition as a temporary setback. George and colleagues found that oral surgery patients who expected post-surgical pain had more reported pain and slower healing than did those patients with high expectations of a rapid recovery.

These and other studies indicate that attitude affects not only the actual physiological rate of recovery, but also the patient's self-reports of pain and post-operative complications (i.e., repeat visits and 2:00 a.m. emergency calls).

Our clinical experience with patients at the Dental Fears Research Clinic illustrates the importance of psychological factors in post-operative recovery. The fearful patient is far more likely to experience difficulties both during and following the appointment than is a non-anxious patient. Those patients with Generalized Anxiety are the most likely to call following treatment with questions or complaints of pain. This may be because of their characteristic tendency to worry. We use two basic strategies to enhance recovery and decrease post-operative complications. The first technique focuses on what can be termed suggestion in the broad sense of the word. The second focuses on cognitive coping techniques that we teach to help the patient deal with the procedure itself as well as the recovery period.

Suggestion and the Role of Information

A lot has been written about how much information one should give patients before and after surgical procedures. Clum (1979) indicated that patients who received additional information experienced more post-operative pain than those who received the usual amount. Other studies tend to confirm that simply giving the patient more information is not effective in preparing him for surgery and, with some patients, may be counterproductive. This is not to say we should avoid providing the patient information, but it points to the fact that it is not sufficient to help him cope optimally with restorative procedures. Research by Schmitt (1973) and George (1980) indicates that working to modify the patient's expectations and attitudes towards the event results in fewer post-operative complications and a more rapid recovery.

As we mentioned previously, we attempt to begin dental treatment with procedures that are less threatening to the patient in order to desensitize him to the dental environment. This allows us to spend time talking with him, preparing for the more feared procedure. This *includes* providing information, but it is used in the context of helping the patient enhance positive expectations towards the event.

It should be remembered that information is a form of "suggestion." Thus, it is important that all communication with the patient be geared towards improving her recovery. A sense of control may be important. For example, suggesting that the patient can take positive actions to speed recovery, such as warm salt water rinses, may provide a sense of control over recovery. Reassurance that help is available, if needed, also may improve acceptance of conditions and mitigates a tendency to worry.

We attempt to help the patient place future appointments in a positive perspective. We find that for many patients, being able to successfully complete work they have long feared and avoided is symbolic of "getting their act together," which they perceive as a significant accomplishment. At every step, we provide positive reinforcement for their progress and encourage their efforts to overcome fears. Immediately before the procedure, we rehearse with the patient the coping techniques to be used, and briefly re-explain what we are going to do during the actual procedure, the rationale behind it, and what we expect will happen immediately following recovery. We provide the most detailed information, not about treatment procedures, but about what to expect during the post-operative period. We try to identify both sensations that are part of the normal recovery and sensations that are abnormal so that patients worry less.

The evening following any treatment, we *routinely* call patients who have a high probability of experiencing post-operative difficulties. These calls reduce the worrying thoughts that many of our patients experience. This technique allows us to contact the patient at *our* convenience and eliminate most late-night calls at home, and it reinforces our efforts at maintaining rapport.

Additionally, we have created a series of short handouts which we give to patients after the appointment. They explain in writing the points that we have discussed verbally.

Coping Strategies

The second major strategy involves teaching the patient cognitive coping techniques. Numerous studies indicate that these are effective in reducing post-operative complications. In a study of 97 abdominal surgery patients, Egbert (1964) found that surgeons could improve patients' recovery by teaching them physical and psychological coping techniques before surgery. Following surgery they rated their pain as less intense, requested less medication, and were discharged earlier than those in the control group. In a study of 25 male patients scheduled for general surgery procedures, Schmitt and Wooldridge (1973) found that the patient group who met with a nurse before surgery to discuss their fears and concerns reported less post-operative pain and was discharged earlier than a comparable control group. Finally, Langer and colleagues (1974) found in a study of 60 patients undergoing general surgery that giving patients a coping device for dealing with post-surgical pain (directing attention to the favorable consequences of their recent surgery) reduced pain reports significantly more than did information alone.

A simple coping technique that is useful during the post-operative recovery period is self-distraction. We encourage the patient to resume normal activities as soon as possible and to read, watch TV, etc. during rest periods rather than lying about focusing on pain. We also tell patients, before surgery, to prepare for a special, relaxing, low-key evening. Another pragmatic technique is to use mental and muscle relaxation instructions, which help patients cope with immediate stress in the operatory as well as during the post-surgical period.

Post-Operative Medications

As explained earlier, the most effective post operative medication is that given as a loading dose before the actual procedure, whether a routine operation or an emergency treatment. If the patient can tolerate an NSAID, it is the drug class of choice for most situations. Dionne (1992) has suggested that ibuprofen (400 mg orally) is particularly effective. Other drugs in this class include flurbiprofen (Ansaid®) or ketorolac tromethamine (Toradol®). Salicyclates, such as aspirin or the longer acting diflunisal (Dolobid®), are also effective. If the patient is unable to take NSAID type drugs, then acetaminophen (paracetemol) should be substituted. When central effects are desired, codeine may be combined with these agents in small amounts. In the U.S.A., combinations of aspirin or acetaminophen and codeine (15 mg, 30 mg) are available by prescription. In other countries, separate prescriptions must be written for the codeine. This is also true when ibuprofen is combined with codeine. Patients should be cautioned when using codeine based medicines that nausea is a common sign of overdose and is often confused with allergy. A phone call to the patient in the post-operative period often serves to check on how much drug a patient is taking and helps avoid overdose. Patients should be told that most dental pain is markedly reduced after 24 hours. If pain does not decrease, see the patient.

SUMMARY

In this chapter we have examined the nature of pain and its relationship to personality, cultural factors, and anxiety. We discussed the use of topical and local anesthetics to enhance pain control and those factors which contribute to anesthetic failure. Finally, we looked at the steps the dentist can take to minimize post-operative pain problems.

QUESTIONS AND EXERCISES

1. Studies have shown that problems with inadequate anesthesia occurs for about _____ percent of patients.

2. Outline the steps the text recommends in achieving anesthesia with a patient who is not fearful of injections and has repeatedly had pain control problems in the mandible.

3. How can you use the research on the relationship between anxiety and pain to your clinical advantage in treating patients?

4. What does research indicate to be the post-operative preparation or information that is most useful in helping patients cope during the recovery period?

EIGHT

Specific Problems

- Needle Phobias
- Gagging
- Adverse Reactions to Local Anesthetic
- Prosthodontics
- Fear of the Dental Environment
- Making Referrals

Introduction

In this chapter we will address some of the more common problems which confront dental professionals in practice. You will see how many of the techniques and strategies previously discussed can be combined and applied to a specific problem. Assessment of the patient's concerns is the key in helping you determine what needs to be done to help him learn to better tolerate treatment. We will also discuss in detail how and when to make referrals to a specialist or other healthcare professional if you determine the patient needs additional services.

NEEDLE PHOBIAS

Patient fear of the needle is one of the most commonly encountered problems in dental practice. What practitioner has not seen a child panic at the sight of a needle? Who hasn't had a patient request that the drilling be done without local anesthetic? And who hasn't seen an adult patient who could tolerate everything but the injection? Because injections are so familiar to us, and because we know that most injections are virtually pain free, it can be difficult to understand a patient's aversion.

We know that most needle fears originate in childhood and usually have resulted from aversive medical or dental experiences. While some patients focus on the pain of the injections, others are panicked by the idea of a sharpened object penetrating the body. Still others can say nothing more about the origin or reasons for their fear beyond the fact they are "just terrified."

How can you best overcome a patient's fears? We believe that it is important to start with a brief assessment of the problem. The following questions are useful:

1. **Do you know how or when your fear of needles began?** You may or may not learn something helpful, but it is a logical starting point of the discussion.

2. **How do you feel about medical injections or blood draws?** This question helps you determine how generalized the problem is. A patient who has few or moderate problems with medical procedures will have minimal

difficulty overcoming a fear of dental injections. On the other hand, if the patient hasn't seen a physician for ten years because "they might want to give me a shot," you face a more difficult challenge.

3. **What is it about injections that is so scary? Is it the pain, the idea of a needle in your body, or something else?** The problem of pain is easy to overcome. Once a patient has a good experience the fear will fade quickly. If the fear is more a result of cognitive upset, it will take more than a "painless injection" to overcome the fear. If the patient relates that it is the anesthetic itself (not the needle), see the section on adverse reactions to local anesthetic later in this chapter.

4. **Imagine that you stuck yourself with a sewing needle, (or safety pin). On a 1-10 scale (10 being the worst) how painful, and how scary, would that be compared to a dental injection?** With this question you are attempting to better understand the patient's tolerance to more everyday unpleasant events compared to his fear of injections. For instance, is he blood phobic, fearful of any type of pain, or just generally fearful?

With adults, the answer to these questions, in addition to an assessment of the patient's overall coping style, should give you enough information to formulate a treatment plan. With children, overcoming a needle fear is somewhat less straightforward, although the basic treatment strategies do not differ. Special considerations for school-age children and adolescents are discussed in Chapter 10.

The fundamental approach to overcoming fear of injections is outlined in Chapter 6 in the section on Practice Strategies. The patient must first be taught basic relaxation skills. Once she has mastered these skills, she is then gradually exposed to the feared stimuli through a series of increasingly realistic and repeated rehearsals. This hierarchy generally begins with an explanation of the basic facts of dental injections and a visual examination of the syringe and needle. It then progresses through repeated practices of the various components of an injection—being leaned back, topical placement, insertion of the syringe with the cap on, insertion with the cap off. It can be helpful to intersperse the practice sessions with some information about what you do to minimize physical discomfort, such as allowing enough time for the topical anesthetic to take effect, injecting very slowly, and using sharp, small-gauge needles. Information does not necessarily reduce fear, but it enhances the patient's sense of cognitive control and helps take away the fear of the unfamiliar or unknown. During each rehearsal coach the patient to practice her breathing and muscle relaxation skills and to use a cognitive coping strategy if she has selected one.

How long does it take to overcome a fear of needles with an adult patient? We have found that it takes about three 45-minute sessions about a week apart to overcome a lifelong fear. While this is a significant block of time, it is a very short time to overcome a severe debilitating problem which interferes with a person's receiving normal dental or medical care.

GAGGING

At some point every dentist, dental hygienist, and dental assistant has been confronted with a gagging patient. Fortunately, in many cases a way is found to "get through" the problem and proceed with treatment. However, there are some patients whose gagging is so severe as to make treatment virtually impossible. Because each of us has a gag reflex, it is easy to view gagging as primarily a physiological problem whose solution avoids stimulating the "sensitive areas." We believe the problem is more accurately viewed as a psychophysiological reaction which has become "over learned." In other words, there is always a significant psychological component. If it is dealt with, the patient's gagging will be reduced to a level where virtually any dental procedure can be successfully completed.

Most gagging patients are quick to tell us of their problem. The vast majority believe that it is an involuntary reaction which they can do nothing about. Consequently, such patients frequently indicate very few fear responses on the assessment scales discussed in Chapter 4. We have learned that the patient's initial self-report about the severity of the problem is frequently not borne out by actual clinical experience. Again, the key to efficient and effective treatment is assessment. Below are questions which we have found helpful.

Interview Questions

1. How did your gagging problem start? How long has it been a problem?

2. What kinds of things make you gag? (Question the patient for dental stimuli such as impressions and radiographs, and non-dental stimuli such as unpleasant odors and stress.)

3. What kinds of problems do you have brushing your teeth? When? What areas?

4. Do you have any problems eating any kind of foods (such as steak)?

5. If you had something caught between your teeth (like popcorn) how would you get it out? Use a toothpick, floss, toothbrush?

6. Can you touch your tongue to the last tooth in the back on the top (bottom)?

The answers to questions 3 to 6 can be very useful in helping you determine to what degree the problem is related to *control*. The activities mentioned above are stimuli controlled by the patient. In most cases they seldom cause the same "reflex" to occur as does stimulation by *someone else* in the same area.

Clinical Assessment

It is also important to perform a clinical assessment of the patient's ability to accept treatment. During your initial exam, begin slowly with a visual exam using the mirror. If the patient appears to tolerate this simple procedure, slowly introduce other intraoral manipulations, simulating those required for treatment. End the exam at the first hint of stimulating the gag response.

Treatment Strategy

The goal of this treatment is to allow the patient to receive care. The objectives are the reduction of anxiety, and the "unlearning" of the thoughts and behaviors that lead to gagging. Systematic desensitization, as described in Chapter 6, treats both of these components simultaneously. Procedurally, the patient is first trained in breathing and muscle relaxation. Next, you identify a graded hierarchy of anxiety or gag-provoking stimuli. Finally, expose the patient sequentially to the items on the list while she is practicing relaxation. The key is to begin with a task which is *just* beyond the patient's current ability to perform.

How do you explain your assessment of the patient's problems, and how you intend to solve it? Let's look at the following conversation:

> Dentist: Thank you for answering all my questions and letting me examine you. I have learned several things. First, it is clear that there are some things which you can do on your own which you can not let others do *to* you. What that tells me is that your gagging problems are not solely a problem of an overly sensitive reflex. That is, the problem varies depending on who is doing what. Does that make sense?

> Patient: Well yeah, I guess.

> Dentist: Let me explain it a little differently. If your gagging was a completely involuntary reflex it wouldn't matter what or who touched the area. Your tongue, a tooth brush, my mirror, or you. *Everything* would trigger it.

> Patient: I do know it's worse at the dentist. I can brush my teeth all right, but I gag whenever the hygienist tries to do something.

> Dentist: Exactly. That tells me that there is a mental, or learning component to your problem. And, if you once learned it, there are some things you can do to "unlearn" it to become less of a gagger. Are you willing to give it a try?

> Patient: Sure. What do I have to lose?

It is crucial to choose a task which is very close to what the patient can *already* do so that he will succeed! One patient may have to begin by placing an index finger on the tooth you wish to x-ray. Another may start by practicing with an empty quadrant tray in preparation for taking a full upper impression. Still another may have to practice with a bite wing placed near the anteriors before being able to move it further back. For example, consider the new patient who needs a full mouth set of radiographs, but says he "can't take x-rays." In assessing what he can and can not do you find that he is able to place his index finger behind both the upper and lower anteriors. Next, you find that he can place a film in the same areas when he holds it place. On the upper jaw he can place a film against the canines. But then on the lower, the same placement appears to initiate a gag response. You should stop at this point. The dentist or assistant might say something like the following.

Assistant: OK. I have found some things that you can tolerate, and some others which are just beyond your abilities.

Patient: Yeah, I started to feel like I was going to gag when I put the tab on the bottom.

Assistant: That's fine. That's just what we were looking for. Over the next week I want you to practice holding your index finger for 10-second periods in that area twice a day as you do your breathing exercises. Once you are comfortable with that, I want you to try placing the film in that area. I also want you to continue to practice placing the film directly behind your front teeth. On the upper jaw where it is easier for you I would like you to try moving the film back one tooth further. (Demonstrate). Any questions?

Patient: How long should I practice for each day?

Assistant: Oh, I forgot to mention that. Each practice session should only be for five to ten minutes. One last thing. If you feel that you are going to gag, just remove your finger or the film, take four to five deep breaths, and once you feel relaxed, begin again. I don't want you to push yourself so that you gag.

We frequently send a patient home with an impression tray, film, or a rubber dam and frame to use for practice. Ask the patient to come back in a week for a 10-minute "progress check." If she makes no progress, problem solve and find a simpler task. If she succeeds give her a new, slightly more difficult assignment. Give the patient praise and encouragement. Because gagging patients are usually motivated they tend to make rapid progress once they are given a method. Most patients learn how to tolerate the required dental procedure within two to six weeks. The best person in the office to work with patients who have this type of problem may be a caring assistant, because she often performs the procedures which elicit gagging in most patients. She should have an interest in helping patients learn new skills, and she needs to become familiar with basic breathing and practice strategies.

What about strategies such as the *temporal tap*, spraying the mouth with topical anesthesias, having the patient "hum" an extended note, or putting salt on the tongue? All of these techniques have been used and all of them work to some degree on some patients. However, we believe that they work *because* they are distracting. If a patient becomes too focused on how his throat feels, whether his tongue is touching the film, or is too worried about doing well for you, his anxiety increases and his ability to tolerate stimulation decreases. Thus, in moderate cases of gagging, a distraction technique will often prove sufficient. Even in more severe cases a full desensitization program may be unnecessary. However, we have found that using graded homework exercises is usually the easiest and most efficient way to overcome a gagging problem.

ADVERSE REACTIONS TO LOCAL ANESTHETICS

The Problem of Adverse Effects with Local Anesthetics

Before discussing adverse effects, a definition is necessary. Evers and Haegerstam (1981) define an adverse effect as an untoward reaction to the administration of local anesthetics including allergic reactions, systemic toxic reactions, psychogenic effects, or drug interactions.

The frequency of adverse effects reported is much higher in dentistry than in medicine. Adverse effects range up to 30 percent of the appointments in which anesthetics are administered. They also differ in type. In medicine they are mostly toxic. In dentistry they appear to be somatic manifestations of fear, which we believe may or may not occur with a cognitive component. Effects include palpitations, dizziness, nausea, tremor, sweating, pallor, and fainting. Interestingly, these effects are similar to systemic reactions to intravenous vasoconstrictor administration. Persson (1969) postulates that adverse effects appearing within one-to-two minutes of injection are likely due to the body's own release of epinephrine rather than to the effects of local anesthetic or vasoconstrictor, although evidence is lacking.

Two large clinical dentistry studies have evaluated local anesthetic reactions. In one double-blind study (Goldman & Gray, 1963) 67 dentists in four different dental settings (hospital, military, dental school, and private practice) reported 12,079 cases involving the use of 3% prilocaine with epinephrine 1:300,000, 2% prilocaine with 1:200,000 epinephrine, and 2% lidocaine with 1:80,000 epinephrine. The overall frequency of side effects was 11.4 percent, a percentage the investigators found unexpectedly high.

In another, more controlled study in which data were collected over a 10-month period, patients received local anesthetics with and without vasoconstrictors (Persson, 1969). The investigator recorded adverse effects in 75 of 2960 cases (2.5 percent). The reports included pallor, nausea, sweating, dizziness, and fainting. The author was unable to associate increased concentrations of vasoconstrictors with increased adverse effects. On the other hand, one study showed an increased percentage of adverse effects with 2% procaine with 1:50,000 epinephrine versus 2% procaine alone for dental student subjects (Costich, 1956).

Evaluation of topical anesthetics has been minimal. Topical anesthetics are administered in order to reduce the pain associated with needle insertion. Theoretically they could reduce adverse effects of the anesthetic caused by anxiety. Improper applications, however, may make their use ineffective. Onset of anesthesia takes from two-to-five minutes, much slower than anesthesia by injection (American Dental Association, 1982). If the procedure is hurried, a resulting painful injection may lead to fear. Many of the preparations are ester-type anesthetics that may cause an allergic reaction. Moreover, some preparations are marketed in pressurized spray containers that are difficult to control, either in dose or site of application. Pollack (1966) postulates that suggestion rather than the topical anesthetic itself may be the critical factor in determining whether the patient feels the placement of the anesthetic needle. Among the subjects receiving topical anesthetic, nearly 69 percent of those told it would not hurt reacted indifferently to the injection, whereas only 58 percent of those receiving no suggestion remained calm. Moreover, when extreme patient reactions did occur, they happened nearly twice as frequently in the control group (6.4 percent) as in the experimental groups (3.7 percent). Results of studies involving topical anesthetics may be difficult to interpret because of the potential occurrence of adverse effects associated with the local anesthetic or the injection procedure itself.

Evidence in the literature suggests that patient characteristics influence local anesthetic adverse effects. Factors hypothesized include fear, previous experience associated with local anesthetics (including being treated without being numb), misattribution of drug effects, medical conditions and drug interactions, drug history, and age (related to fear) and gender.

Patients who fear local anesthetics often focus their attention on their bodies. Just as patients with general anxiety cannot manage to control their fearful thoughts, these patients are preoccupied with bodily sensations, usually intense, that gives them the opportunity for misinterpretation and misattribution. Knowledge of the patient's focus of attention is the key to successful diagnosis and treatment.

Some patients' fear is the fear response itself—the panic of "being out of control" emotionally. Most, however, are anxious that they will experience a dangerous physical reaction. These patients may be afraid of a catastrophe such as a stroke, heart attack, or choking to death. They may be convinced that they are allergic to lidocaine or epinephrine, or that dentist error or even a standard dental treatment will result in severe injury or death. Ironically, though stricken with panic, many do not think of themselves as being fearful. They may deny fear or see it as secondary. They are often capable of discussing their body problems in a very logical and thoughtful manner. However, they are very often resistant to changing how they view their problem and present a serious challenge to the clinician.

The problem usually centers on fear of a specific procedure, agent, or sensation. Fear of adverse effects from local anesthetics is not uncommon. Other problems include the sensation of numbness itself, fear of choking with a rubber dam or other dental device, and sensitivity to other dental drugs and materials.

A patient's history with local anesthetic may predict future adverse effects. Persson (1969) noted that one percent (30/2960) of his subjects had more than once before experienced general side reactions to local anesthetic. Of this total, 40 percent subsequently reported at least one adverse effect during the course of the study. Goldman and Gray (1963) reported that five percent of 12,079 cases had a history of adverse effects, which were not enumerated. Another example of previous experience with local anesthetic involves patients being treated without profound anesthesia. Persson (1969) found that 14 percent (372/2960) of his cases with adverse effects had only partial or unsuccessful anesthesia. Partial anesthesia was defined as there being some pain during the procedure not requiring a supplementary dose of anesthetic. Unsuccessful anesthesia required one or more supplementary doses. The overall percentage of adverse effects with complete anesthesia was two percent (57/2558). However, partial anesthesia resulted in four percent (14/318) having side effects and unsuccessful anesthesia seven percent (4/54). We do not know whether being treated while not numb was considered to be a previous adverse reaction to local anesthetic in this study. Nor is it known how many of the 372 reporting incomplete anesthesia had a previous history of failure to get numb. In a recent survey of an insured dental population (Weinstein *et al.*, 1985), 60 percent of subjects reporting anesthetic failure at their last dental visit also reported previous difficulty in getting numb. Kaufmann and colleagues (1984) reported a high percentage of dental anxiety (47 percent) among patients with a history of failure to get numb. Milgrom and colleagues (1984) suggest that this anxiety may lead to further anesthetic failure, resulting in mismanagement by the dentist and inappropriate use of local anesthetics. This in turn may lead to further adverse effects.

The reported incidence of true local anesthetic allergies is extremely low (VanArsdel, 1984). Nonetheless, patients are frequently advised that adverse reactions experienced during injections are allergic in nature and that they should avoid particular anesthetic solutions. DeShazo and Nelson (1979) allergy tested 90 patients referred with the diagnosis of lidocaine allergy, including 14 having a history of immediate hypersensitivity reaction. Not one of the 90 proved hypersensitive when skin tested and challenged with increasing concentrations of the drug. In a similar study, Babajews and lvanyi (1982) found only three patients out of 37 reporting previous untoward reactions to be allergic. Aldrete and Johnson (1970) surveyed 809 incidents of drug reaction. Allergies were found in 525 cases, but local anesthetic could be implicated only three times. Other drugs with frequent adverse reactions are also subject to mislabeling as allergies. Allergic rashes associated with ampicillin constitute only one third of the rashes seen accompanying this drug (Geyman & Erickson, 1978). Yet patients are frequently taken off the drug unnecessarily and advised to avoid ampicillin and other penicillins in the future. Moreover, VanArsdel (1982) reports that patients with known penicillin allergies can frequently be treated successfully with the drug within two years of their last reaction. He estimates that five out of six patients with positive testing of penicillin allergy can safely receive the antibiotic.

Mislabeling of adverse drug reactions may lead to more expensive and/or less effective treatment alternatives. For example, Malamed (1973) has recommended diphenhydramine as a substitute for people reported allergic to local anesthetics. This antihistamine, however, is known to be less effective as a local anesthetic in terms of duration and quality of anesthesia and may cause pain during injection. This may lead to elevated fear levels and increased adverse effects. Other alternatives such as general anesthesia or IV sedation may prove unacceptable because of cost or increased medical risk, leading to patients' avoidance of treatment and worsening of dental problems. In short, because of misunderstanding or not knowing the cause of local anesthetic adverse effects, dentists themselves may be contributing to the increased frequency of untoward effects.

Dentist Variables

Dentist variables relate to what the dentist does during injections based upon his beliefs, knowledge, and experience. It is important to consider communication with the patient, length of injection time, use of aspirating syringes, and drug knowledge.

Studies of dental fear have shown that dentist behavior and communication skills are important etiologic factors (Smith *et al.*, 1984). Providing clear explanations, taking adequate time so the patient does not feel rushed, listening to patient concerns, and the credibility of what the dentist says have been shown to reduce pain (Dangott *et al.*, 1978) and may influence the incidence of local anesthetic adverse effects. Injecting too rapidly may cause pain and elevate fear levels. Moreover, patient apprehension may increase with prolonged waiting time between injections when supplemental doses are required. Kaufman and colleagues (1984) suggest that increased volumes of anesthetics be used at the outset, with supplementary doses to follow if signs of anesthesia do not appear within one to two minutes. The use of aspirating syringes has been recommended by the American Dental Association Council on Dental Materials and Devices, which notes that positive aspirations of blood were reported among 2.6 to 30 percent of inferior alveolar injections in different series of patients (Alling & Christopher, 1974). A positive aspiration means that the point of the needle is either in a vessel or in a pool of blood. Failure to move the needle away from this area may lead to intravascular injections and toxicity. Traeger (1979) suggests that a hematoma resulting from such an accident may provide one reason for anesthetic failures, particularly within the inferior alveolar nerve site. In addition, Oikarinen *et al.* (1975) demonstrated that needle gauge is an unimportant factor in eliciting pain during injections.

Dentists' beliefs concerning local anesthetics may be a function of early training in dental school. There the student is taught very little about either recognizing or treating systematic fear (Milgrom *et al.*, 1984). Fiset and Weinstein (1983) have demonstrated that dentists may not attend to all of their patients' verbal and non-verbal indications of distress. Therefore, local adverse effects may be misattributed to the drug rather than to some other factor relating to the patients themselves, resulting in misuse of drugs and mismanagement of the patients, which may lead to further adverse effects.

Patients with Agoraphobia or Panic Disorder

Some patients who report that they are physically responsive in the dental environment have a history of agoraphobia or panic disorder; their problem receiving dental care is part of a larger problem. Agoraphobics, usually women, have a high level of general anxiety and often depression as well. They describe a diffuse set of fears including fear of passing out, having a heart attack, being trapped, losing control, or "going crazy." They describe aversive physical sensations before and while leaving what they believe to be the safety of their home or elsewhere or when their trusted companion is not readily available. Agoraphobics avoid places they believe to be unsafe. They are not frightened *per se* by being in a crowded shopping mall, bus, or grocery store; they are concerned that they may not be safe in such environments and that they may have an aversive or dangerous episode that might put them in the hospital, or worse. There is some evidence that the majority of agoraphobics have a history of panic attacks and that their phobic avoidance is a function of the circumstances of previous panic attacks.

A trusted companion reduces danger and assures some level of physical safety for these people. The issue of being safe is central to their willingness to enter new environments. For agoraphobics, dental offices and clinics are not inherently safe. They believe that dental personnel do not know what to do in medical or psychiatric emergencies. Moreover, the patient may fear embarrassment .

Patients who report agoraphobic or panic disorder symptoms should not be treated by dental personnel without the consultation of a psychiatrist or psychologist. Referral before treatment is very desirable. Even with competent treatment, the core fear—that they are not safe—is not often completely removed. Agoraphobics will have some residual fear even after psychotherapy. Many never completely accept that something terrible will not happen to them. Because they may believe that there is something wrong with their bodies, many can never completely accept the fact that dental treatment presents no special risks for them.

Panic Disorders and Biological Explanations

Research by David Sheehan (1980, 1982) and others indicates that frightening though minor medical conditions such as heart pounding, tachycardia, light-headedness, nausea, rubbery legs, choking sensations, etc., may be caused by an underlying bio-chemical abnormality or cardiovascular pathology (mitral valve prolapse) and are responsible for some cases of panic disorders. This has been categorized as endogenous anxiety. Exogenous anxiety, on the other hand, is focused on external events and is usually said to be limited to specific settings.

Recently Weiner and Sheehan (1990) surveyed over 400 people regarding both dental and other fearful situations, symptoms, and complaints and found that the presence of spontaneous panic attacks differentiated subjects into endogenous/exogenous groupings. The researchers believe that endogenous anxiety is a medical disorder that mimics ordinary anxiety and should be treated through drugs such as alprazolam, phenelzine, or imipramine. While the data presented by this study are well accepted, the conclusion is controversial (Roy-Byrne *et al.*, 1994). Biological theories of panic disorders have been subject to a number of criticisms.

Our view is that whether or not panic-related disorders have a biological component in their etiology, it is clear that conditioning is extremely important.

In our clinical experience, we have found that patients can be taught to "decondition" themselves by learning to identify initial symptoms such as hyperventilation or tachychardia that allow them to short circuit the panic reaction in its early phases.

Patients Without Agoraphobia or Panic Disorder: The Problem of Misattribution

Most patients who report a physical response to dental treatment do not have a history of agoraphobia or panic disorder. At present, diagnosis of Panic Disorder requires frequent attacks with multiple physical symptoms (four times in four weeks), at least one of which was unexpected (*DSM-IV*,1994). Moreover, most of our patients who focus their attention on bodily symptoms do not fear an inability to escape or lack control in other than dental settings. Our experience has taught us that the fear of a medical catastrophe or panic that these non-psychiatric patients show is the result of catastrophic misinterpretation of bodily sensations, a decidedly psychological explanation similar in most ways to the views of Clark (1988) on the etiology of panic disorders. On the other hand, although the problem is cognitive in nature patients are resistant to reinterpretations of the meaning of sensations thought to herald danger.

Origin of the Fear

There are two complementary psychological conceptualizations that help explain how a person experiencing dental fear becomes emotionally upset. They are especially useful in understanding patients who are afraid of catastrophe related to local anesthetics. The first theory is outlined as follows:

Environmental stimulus → physiological arousal → upset

The patient who has gone regularly to the dentist and unexpectedly has an intense, frightening experience, with a pounding heart and nausea is an example. The stimulus of the injection itself or anesthetic numbness results in arousal. Negative thoughts about the significance of those sensations lead to upset and panic. Simply put, the theory behind this formulation claims: *The emotions we experience depend on the label we place on the arousal felt inside our bodies.*

The second conceptualization looks at the upset of patients as follows:

Environmental stimulus → negative thoughts → physiological arousal → upset

In the second theory, an environmental stimulus, e.g., a rubber dam, leads to negative thoughts ("I won't be able to breathe" or "I'll choke"), followed by physiological arousal (which is triggered by difficulty swallowing), and an extreme panic response.

In 1962, Schachter and Singer conducted a classic experiment that has greatly influenced how psychologists view emotions. They administered epinephrine by injection to a subject who was told that it was Suproxin, a new vitamin compound. The subject was then placed in a waiting room for 15 to 20 minutes. A stooge, supposedly just Suproxin injected, was brought in to pass the waiting time with the subject. A short while after the injection, the subject experienced typical nervous system arousal: hand tremors, heart pounding, and rapid breathing. As the drug took effect, the stooge began behaving in one of two ways. He either became progressively angry or increasingly euphoric. During this period, the investigators watched the subject through a two-way mirror and observed and systematically recorded his behavior. They found that subjects who had waited with the angry stooge became angry, and those who waited with the euphoric stooge became euphoric. Subjects with a saline placebo had no emotional reaction, no matter how the stooge functioned. Subjects who were warned in advance that Suproxin sometimes will have side effects like trembling and heart pounding had no emotional reaction, regardless of the stooge's behavior.

Schachter drew the following conclusions from the experiment:

1. Emotion is not merely a chemical reaction that automatically creates feelings. Physiological arousal, by itself, cannot produce specific emotions.

2. A state of physiological arousal for which the subject has no immediate explanation makes him want to understand it. He will actively search his environment for an appropriate explanation or "label" for the arousal. Choice of labels will determine the emotional response.

A specific emotion is, at least in part, created by our evaluation of internal and external events. Subjects in the study attributed their arousal to either anger or euphoria depending on what appeared to be appropriate, based on the emotional reaction of the stooge.

Schacter's study has important implications for treating emotional upset. It suggests that patients become anxious, for example, by saying certain things to themselves. They attribute their physiological arousal to the emotion of fear and consequently interpret something in their environment as implying danger. They can make this interpretation by seeing something that seems threatening or noticing that someone else is afraid and believing that there must be good reason for alarm. *Emotion depends on thought.* Thought precedes emotion. If the attributions and interpretations can be changed, so can the distressing emotion. Health professionals influence these thoughts. For example, there are clinical reports of fearful patients who, when told that arousal (e.g., increased heart beat) was caused by the epinephrine in the anesthetic and not their fear, became much less fearful. On the other hand, it is our impression that clinicians often attribute fear-related responses to drug reactions.

Cognitive theorists Beck (1979) and Ellis (1975) are the leading proponents of the second theory. They argue that emotional reactions are a result of the way we structure reality. They suggest that if patients are anxious, it is because they are interpreting events as dangerous. If a patient is depressed, it is because he sees himself as defective or the victim of loss. His anger is produced by perceptions that he is suffering from abuse and is a victim of injustice. *Each painful emotion is created by a particular negative thought.*

Chronic upset is the by-product of a systematic bias in viewing the world. To the "depressive," for example, every event is an opportunity to see himself in some way diminished. Then he gets the "sinking feeling" in his stomach, which he labels depression. The anxious person tends to view even innocuous events as threatening. Many of our patients fear even the rubber prophy cup. These threats set off the "fight or flight" alarm responses, which he labels anxiety.

These two theories of emotion indicate the importance of patient thought in the fear response. The theories are complementary and both help to explain the behavior of our patients in this diagnostic category—those who misattribute the source of their problem. These theories are important to you as a clinician in understanding how to work with such patients. The patient has a role too; he is not just a victim of previous conditioning. The way he labels or evaluates the situation in the future determines his emotional reactions. The dentist, in treating the fear, can help the patient learn to recognize the fear reaction for what it is—an unpleasant yet not dangerous situation.

Providing Treatment

Providing treatment to patients with fear of adverse or aversive physiological responses involves two steps that are linked. First it is necessary to establish trust, and then it is necessary to alter attribution.

Establishing Trust and Safety: the Diagnosis

Patients need to trust the professional judgment of the dentist; the patient must be convinced that the dentist is extremely competent in his diagnostic ability and can provide a safe environment if his worst fears are realized. A patient will discount a quick answer to his problem, especially if he believes the proper "solution" places him at risk.

Students and inexperienced clinicians tend to reassure these patients prematurely. Such reassurance ("Don't worry, it's only anxiety") is not effective and serves to deny or discredit legitimate patient concerns. Paradoxically, to establish trust and credibility with the patient we indicate that *we take the problem seriously*. We carefully gather information before making a differential diagnosis. We take a detailed dental and medical history. We write to or call dentists, physicians, or others who know previous events in the patient's history. The history you take should be thorough. Contact subject matter experts and read and copy relevant scientific articles.

Fiset and colleagues (1985) suggest that for local anesthesia-related adverse reactions the history should include the nature, time of onset, and duration of all reactions the patient has experienced. Drug information should include the type, concentration, number of cartridges administered, type of vasoconstrictor, the site of administration, and whether a topical was used. Other information that is helpful in reconstructing the adverse event(s) includes medications the patient took concurrently, sedative agents provided by the dentist and others, fear of injections and other dental fears, psychiatric history, and chair positioning (to help determine whether a syncopal reaction occurred).

The most probable cause of the patient's reactions will emerge when all of the data áre collected and studied. Differential diagnoses include psychophysiological response, systemic toxicity, and allergic reaction. While almost all adverse responses are psychophysiological, it is critical not to skip the differential diagnosis.

A conversation with a patient who told her new dentist that she had a history of "very scary" reactions to local anesthetic at another dental office might go something like this:

Patient: ... and that's what happened to me. Can you help me?

Dentist: This a serious problem; one that I cannot solve right now. With your permission I am going to gather as much information as I can from everyone involved. I would like you to sign a few releases so I can contact your present physician and your previous dentist.

Patient: Okay. But this seems like a lot of trouble for you.

Dentist: It is important to get at the root of this problem and

> to find a way to treat you that is both safe and
> efficacious. In fact, depending on what I learn from
> my contact wi th your doctors, I may even advise
> you to be allergy tested or may place you in the
> dental chair and do some tests myself.

At times, sending the patient to an allergist for testing is necessary, not so much to rule out allergies or sensitivities, but to help convince the patient of your thoroughness and the safety of your recommendations. A few words of advice: do not let the patient or the patient's physician choose the allergist. Instead, carefully select and then contact him or her to discuss the patient's problem. Give the allergist information about the drugs he will test. Many allergists recommend avoiding a drug, even when test results are negative. This normal practice by allergists would be a disaster for your efforts to alter attribution.

Altering Attribution

The second step in treating these patients involves altering their perception of the problem. To explain this, let us look at a problem involving an adverse reaction to local anesthetic. It is not uncommon for a patient or the dentist to attribute a reaction to a drug. Patients tell us that they have had adverse reactions to the epinephrine in the anesthetic. Dentists are often convinced and convince these patients that the source of the problem is drug related.

In the simplest clinical case, when an adverse effect just occurs and the patient is not scared and trusts you, it is possible to explain to the patient the real cause of his heart palpitations and give him informational control over the events at the dentist. Imagine this interaction:

Dentist: The anesthetic drug we are using has some normal
side effects you need to understand.

Patient: OK.

Dentist: Mainly you may feel your pulse quicken or even
some chest pounding for a few moments.

Patient: Is this dangerous?

Dentist: No, it is normal and will pass very soon.

With a patient who is afraid of a drug reaction, but trusts you, you may want a different attribution strategy, where you attribute the reaction to normal physiological responses:

Dentist: Have you noticed when you think about receiving an injection that you begin to sweat?

Patient: Yes.

Dentist: This is a normal physiological response to feeling anxious.

Patient: I am worried that I am having a reaction to the drug.

Dentist: The drugs we use have almost no side effects. What you feel should be interpreted as related to anxiety, not drugs.

Although you should attempt such simple explanations, they may not be sufficient to alter patient fear-related responses, especially for patients who do not recognize that they are fearful. For these patients, after we gather data and provide a differential diagnosis, we provide the "broken toaster message" to establish that we understand their problem. It goes something like this:

I know you must feel like a person who has placed a piece of bread in a toaster and almost was electrocuted. Sparks flying everywhere. You take the toaster to an expert ... the small appliance repairman ... and he checks it out with his instruments and tells you that everything is really okay. What do you do? Do you dare use the toaster again? Just because he did not find anything wrong does not mean the situation is not dangerous.

Most patients understand the metaphor, and greatly appreciate the empathy that you generate at this point. It will allow you to proceed: the next step involves a careful examination of the "toaster" by both of you.

DO NOT CHANGE THE ANESTHETIC

It is important that you do *not* recommend changing anesthetic agents. While changing drugs appears to be a rational and quick way to solve the patient's problem, our experience indicates that it has negative results. First, it provides "evidence" to show the patient that you believe that she can not tolerate the drug. She will most likely never again be willing to allow the use of that drug (usually lidocaine with epinepherine). And, if you take out the epinepherine you are likely to hurt her (Fiset *et al.*, 1986). Further, because the problem is anxiety-related, it is not uncommon to find that the patient develops an adverse response to the new drug that you are using!

Case Example

Mr. Green feared that the effect of his panic would be death in the dental chair. He searched out the emergency oxygen in the operatory and repeatedly asked about emergency precautions. He presented with severe periodontal disease and some broken restorations. Our primary strategy involved structuring his visits so that we could do short procedures successfully and providing rest breaks to give him control over the pace of treatment. He often felt the need to sit up after an injection. When more than one injection was required, we programmed rest breaks in between the injections. These rest breaks allowed Mr. Green to use his coping skills to "calm down" and reduce his physiological arousal level before proceeding further—thus reducing his fears "that things will begin to run out of control."

It is important to note that we do not deny that patients experience their particular physical reaction. Instead, we praise them for surviving even though they felt physical upset. These patients will frequently deny that their coping techniques are working and repeatedly need help in learning to control the reaction that they fear will snowball into panic. We tell the patient that his task is to learn to recognize the initial symptoms indicating that he is about to have a "reaction" and use his coping skill to break the chain of events early or at least let the panic pass quickly, with minimal upset.

In more difficult cases, we try to demonstrate that we can recreate such symptoms as tachycardia or dyspnea in the dental environment, without any dental treatment. This helps to demonstrate concretely to the patient that there is a direct connection between his thoughts and physiological reactions. For many this is an important revelation, and helps them learn to control something they once thought was beyond their conscious control. We place the patient in the dental chair and attach a biofeedback monitor, usually a pulse rate monitor that is worn on the earlobe. After some relaxation and breathing instruction, we have the patient imagine the fearful situation. If he remains calm we will do a full rehearsal of an injection. The patient usually becomes aware at this point that the problem is *not* strictly physical. We explain that his re-creation of the feared response is a function of "psychophysiological conditioning," which we will attempt to alter together. We consider this procedure to be part of our differential diagnosis and not treatment. The following case history involving a drug reaction illustrates this point:

Case Example

Mrs. Smith, a healthy 40-year-old mother and a health professional herself, came to us seeking help with her suspected adverse reactions to local anesthetic. She reported that reactions began five years before while she was being treated at her dentist's office. She reported that the reactions began 20 minutes after injection and were characterized by "tachycardia and a drop in blood pressure." The most recent episode resulted in the emergency involvement of a physician, who told her she had reacted to the epinephrine in the anesthetic. The patient subsequently had tests for allergy to the anesthetic and preservative: results were negative.

Mrs. Smith did not appear fearful. On the other hand, she reported that her life is hectic. Her husband noted that she appeared "shaky" a few days before dental visits. As part of our workup we easily determined that she had difficulty accepting the fact that she is not in danger from the anesthetic. She sat vertically in the dental chair and clipped on the lead from a pulsemeter with a digital readout. After a resting heart rate in the mid-70s was established, we asked her to visualize successively making a dental appointment, approaching the dental office, and being seated in the dental chair. Her heart rate rose from the mid-70s to the mid-80s when she visualized making an appointment, and went up and stayed in the mid-90s when she visualized approaching and being seated in the dentist's office. At that point we asked her to "relax." Her response was that her heart rate rose to over 130 bpm and she reported hot flashes and feeling "flushed and panicky." Subsequent discussion revealed a family history of heart disease, and that for Mrs. Smith certain thoughts and situations triggered a panic-like response mimicking a heart attack. With these insights, Mrs. Smith was able to begin to accept a diagnosis that her mind influenced her physiology. We could now begin a treatment giving her control over her physiological reaction.

After the patient recognizes the role of thought in his physiological response to dental treatment, we use one of two treatment modalities in our clinic: a graduated controlled exposure technique or biofeedback (see Chapter 6). These techniques will work with many types of somatic reaction.

A word or two about gradual exposure with local anesthetics are in order: We give the patient very small, subclinical doses of local anesthetic at first, and then progress over appointments to clinical doses. The patient is required to use a coping technique to control arousal and remains in the clinic hooked up to either a pulsemeter for a few hours after the injection. Preoperative and follow-up blood pressure and vital signs are monitored. The patient is never left alone. Patients perceive that this exposure-based treatment, comparable to desensitizations to bee or other insect antigens, is safe and makes good sense. In addition, we ask the patient to call us if she experiences any unusual response. At times, we call the patient to be sure that she is not misattributing a cold or other benign physical symptom to an adverse effect of the drug we used. The case of Mrs. Smith discussed above illustrates how biofeedback can be used to help patients who fear catastrophe, in this case allergic reaction to lidocaine.

She accepted the fact that her response was induced not by the anesthetic but by her fearful reaction to dental treatment. We used the pulsemeter, which functioned very well as an assessment tool, as the major vehicle of her treatment. The goal was to identify and have her practice a response that would take the place of her anxiety. After instructions and a short session of practice she was given the assignment of practicing lowering her heart rate 15 minutes every day.

She recorded in a daily log the time she spent with the device, her heart rate, and subjective responses. After identifying a way to maintain her heart rate at the lowest possible point, she imagined stressful dental and non-dental scenes while she practiced her "calming" response, which relied heavily on control of her respiration. At week four, she was given, in the context of providing dental treatment, half a carpule of anesthetic, with epinephrine. Mrs. Smith, with pulsemeter attached, responded to the placement of the topical anesthetic gel with a 50-beat-per-minute increase in her heart rate to over 140 bpm. She noted that this was just like the previous episode in her dentist's office. Two subsequent appointments for restorative dentistry were uneventful, with the exception of one period of upset with increased heart rate just about 20 minutes after the injection. Mrs. Smith pointed out to us that she was still somewhat conditioned to respond anxiously. At this point she had an insight about why her reaction occurred 20 minutes after the injection. This was about the time her old dentist returned to the operatory to begin treatment. Mystery solved!

PROSTHODONTICS

Denture failures are rarely the result of technical or mechanical faults alone and are seldom corrected by remaking the denture (Winkler, 1989). When a patient is dissatisfied it is likely that the psychological aspects of the treatment were not attended to sufficiently either before or after denture construction.

The Psychology of Loss

Fearful patients who require dentures present special problems to the clinician. When patients face the loss of all of their natural teeth it is not unusual for guilt and depression to overcome them. The loss of the teeth and receiving a denture are frequently perceived as major life events. For a significant minority, tooth loss can symbolize personal defeat, a sign of old age, or a step nearer to death. This can impair acceptance of the treatment plan, or the new denture. A majority of Swedish patients perceived this event as more important in terms of adjustment than events such as marriage, retirement, or changing work (Bergendal, 1989).

Thus, for many people this loss is perceived as akin to amputations, hysterectomies, and mastectomies. Some people do not fare very well after such surgeries. For the most part they had pre-existing psychiatric problems. Knowledge of such conditions is very valuable, because it precludes being surprised when one is faced with adjustment problems and allows you to plan whatever is necessary to help the patient be successful. Clearly, the treatment of such patients requires planning for additional visits and considerable patience and social support.

It is important for the entire dental staff to be not only non-judgmental but supportive. Focus attention on the future, not on the past. Discuss the benefits realistically and reinforce the idea that the patient will have a natural smile and dentition that is functional. Immediate dentures will be appreciated by many patients who fear being without teeth.

The Process of Denture Making and Adjustment

Communication. As Swoope noted in 1973, there are three main objectives in communicating with denture patients: 1) identifying problems early, 2) planning treatment to meet the patient's needs, and 3) preparing the patient carefully. Give the patient examples of the fears and anticipated problems of other patients and ask him how he feels about the anticipated loss or change. Identify the patient's beliefs, expectations and requirements as well. For example, some patients expect that after a denture is fitted they will not have to return for dental care—that dentures are a ticket to a future without dentistry. These and other unrealistic expectations must be addressed during the treatment planning phase.

Planning and choice. The patient's involvement in the design and esthetics of the denture or other appliance is essential to making sure he accepts the final product. Passive acceptance of the clinicians decisions regarding issues such as color, tooth size, and placement may result in subsequent dissatisfaction that is not easily resolved. Old photos of the patient's smile are helpful at times, as are the input from relatives and friends who must "face" him daily. It is a good idea to involve a significant other in the planning and even in the subsequent adjustment process. Many patients require considerable time to psychologically adjust to and accept dentures. We take every caution to avoid rushing through this phase, and frequently use wax up and multiple "try ins" before any final decisions are made.

Adjustment. Difficulties in adapting to the sensations of the new appliance are very common. We have also found that it is much easier for most patients to successfully adapt to one denture at a time. In addition to discomfort with the appliance itself, many patients are ill-prepared to function with a denture.

We stress that a denture is made in phases and requires numerous adjustments as it is "tried in" and used over time. We emphasize that the patient should expect that it will take some time to adjust to the appliance and the compromises in function and feeling that it presents. The problem seems to be worse for patients who lacked a number of teeth for a long period of time. Many patients are surprised to learn that oral hygiene is still important!

Case Example

One of our patients, Kathy, a 42-year-old divorcee employed as a telemarketer, was extremely pleased when her immediate dentures were delivered. However, she was in tears a week later when she reported difficulty eating and speaking and believed people were staring at her because of her dentures. At this appointment we provided a lesson in eating with dentures by instructing Kathy to take only small pieces of food and to balance food between dentures. We provided supervised practice with a banana and coffee cake. We also instructed Kathy to practice eating and to read books aloud to her daughter at home. Kathy agreed to keep a log of the food she ate and her reading. We negotiated an agreement specifying where she would wear her dentures. Kathy returned with her log once a week to have a month for a brief consultation and problem solving session. The approach was successful. While self-conscious, Kathy slowly began to venture into the world with her new dentures and the support of clinic staff.

FEAR OF THE DENTAL ENVIRONMENT

Many patients have concerns about the health risks associated with some technical or procedural aspect of dental care. For example we have all heard scare stories about the danger of amalgams, or the spread of AIDS through dental treatment. In extreme cases these fears form the basis of the catastrophic worries which we have discussed earlier. However, in most situations information and explanation will be sufficient to answer a patient's questions and provide the necessary reassurance. In this section we will look at some of the most common fears about dental treatment and the approach you might take to address your patients' concerns.

Radiographs

Some patients express reluctance to submit to routine radiographs as a result of media exposes about "unnecessary" x-rays. We recommend that you not take radiographs before a patient sees the dentist, or before she is given a clear explanation of their purpose. It is important to reinforce that films are crucial to good diagnosis. Acknowledge the legitimacy of a patient's reluctance by stating that it is your policy to avoid radiographs except when they are needed for accurate assessment of a problem. Take the initiative by explaining safety precautions such as the cervical collar and vest. Have a well practiced answer to the more inevitable questions such as, "How much radiation do I really get?"

An approach such as this should allay the concern of all but the most anxious patients. If a patient refuses necessary radiographs in these circumstances, recognize that there is a serious psychological problem which needs to be addressed. Remember that patients can not legally consent to negligent care.

Amalgam Replacement

Sensational articles about mercury and "silver" fillings occur regularly in the lay press. Many patients, especially those who are interested in nutrition, natural foods, or vitamins will ask questions, or express concern about whether amalgams are dangerous. How should you respond to a patient? Begin by acknowledging that with all the contradictory information we read and hear it is sometimes difficult to sort things out. Tell the patient that you are glad that she asked, and that you are happy to tell her about recent findings in the scientific literature. For example, you might say:

> Amalgams have been the subject of a lot of recent studies. Researchers have found that the amount of mercury in individuals with silver filings is actually lower than in those who eat fish regularly but who have no fillings. And those levels are far below the ones set by the Food and Drug Administration. The American Dental Association has reviewed the evidence and concluded that it is unethical to remove amalgams and replace them with composite fillings and imply that there is any health benefit without consultation with an allergist and tests which show sensitivity to metal. It's also important to realize that plastic or composite fillings have a short life span, and require repeated replacement. The risks of composite also include tooth sensitivity and can result in root canal treatment. The air pollution of most urban areas presents a much more measurable and documented threat to our health than any evidence we have of the effects of amalgam fillings. I have amalgam fillings in my own mouth and believe they are safe.

AIDS

A third area of frequent concern is about infectious diseases, especially AIDS. Many patients hold misconceptions about AIDS and how it is actually spread. We recently saw a new patient in the DFRC who was an admitted "disease phobic." She took elaborate daily precautions, but recognized that her behavior was obsessive. Initially it appeared that it might be impossible to work with her as she complained about the inadequate asepsis of other dental offices. However, she made it clear that information was very helpful and could make a difference in her beliefs and behavior. While she presented an extreme situation we found that the same approach we typically use with patients expressing similar concerns was effective with her.

Begin by acknowledging that some of the routine protection procedures can be somewhat intimidating. Glaros and Gadbury-Amyot (1993) found that college educated patients had more negative emotional reactions to pictures of properly protected dentists than to those dentists who wore no such protection. Second, take time to explain the reasons for your barrier and sterilization techniques— why you wear masks and gloves, why the dental equipment is covered in disposable plastics, and the sterilization procedures for your instruments. Emphasize that your policy is to treat each patient as if she is an active disease carrier in order to protect both you and your patients. Finally, have available some patient oriented brochures which explain infectious diseases and the precautions which dental health professionals take to prevent problems.

There are, however, a few patients whose fears you can not calm. They may seem to ask the same questions or make the same statements following your explanation as they did before you began. Their ideas appear more like beliefs—dearly held and unshakable by reason or information. In such situations we have found that there is often little that can be done. Don't compromise your standard of care for their beliefs. While you can not get into professional difficulties for refusing to violate accepted treatment standards, you can certainly be held liable if you provide such substandard treatment.

MAKING REFERRALS

To this point we have discussed recognizing, assessing, and strategies appropriate for treating various types of dental fears in your practice. Although we have mentioned that in some situations referring a patient to another professional is advised, we have not discussed much about how best to facilitate a successful referral. Experience has taught us that there is a big difference between *making* a referral, having it "stick," and having it turn out to be a positive and useful experience for the patient.

Making a Referral to Another Dentist

There are two different circumstances in which you might make a referral to another dentist. The first, and by far the most common, is when you determine that the patient's dental condition warrants treatment by a specialist such as an endodontist or periodontist. It is probably safe to say that most people needing such services have problems which are a result of years of dental neglect. For many of these patients, fear has been the root of their inattention and avoidance. If your goal is to help this person enter treatment, complete necessary care, and become a regular patient, you should keep in mind several factors. As we have mentioned in our discussion of dental emergencies, and in the section on treatment planning, it is easy to focus on the patient's emergent problems rather than on the goal of ensuring that he has several non-traumatic and successful experiences during the initial visits. Consequently, we recommend that whenever possible, referrals to a specialist be delayed until the patient has undergone some simpler, more straightforward treatment with you. Most dental problems requiring the services of a specialist have developed over a long period, and treatment can be postponed until you have established a successful working relationship with the patient and have completed some simpler procedures with the judicious use of pain medications, antibiotics, or palliative treatment. Once you are ready to make the referral, it is important to have a detailed conversation with the specialist, or to write her a comprehensive letter outlining the patient's history, and what you have done to help this patient overcome his concerns about treatment. It is important to tell the other dentist what has worked to help the patient become less fearful. Be sure to recommend specialists who share your beliefs about treating fearful patients, lest a referral undo all of your investment in the patient.

It is important to keep in mind that if the patient is "too scared" to follow through with the referral, or finds the treatment experience traumatic, he is likely to decide not to return to you or the specialist out of shame, embarrassment, or anger.

The second circumstance for a referral is when you find that the patient is too fearful for you to work with. As dental care providers, all of us tend to choose the kinds of cases we feel comfortable treating. If you see a fearful patient whose fears are beyond what you want to tackle, you may know a colleague who you believe may be more skilled or interested in working with such people. In such circumstances it is best to be straightforward with the patient. Tell him that you want him to succeed in treatment and that your colleague is more skilled in working with people who have problems like his.

This raises a question. How do you determine when the referral should be to a fellow dentist and when it should be to a mental health specialist? A general rule of thumb is this: We all know colleagues who are especially good at some aspect of the dental profession. We might say to ourselves, "If my mom had to have a 5-unit bridge, I'd recommend George J." Or, "If anyone could handle that little girl, it would be Susan H." If you see a fearful patient and you can't imagine *anyone* you know being able to work with him, it is probably appropriate to discuss a referral for psychological services with the patient.

Talking to the Patient's Physician About Mental Health Status

Every dentist has referred patients to a physician to have a medical condition such as diabetes or a heart murmur ruled out before beginning dental treatment. Most of us are much less comfortable talking to a physician about the patient's psychological status. The patient's primary physician in many cases is not the best person with whom to initiate a referral about these matters. However, there are situations where it may be appropriate to discuss the matter first with the patient's physician: in small or rural communities; in situations where the patient has a strong relationship with his physician; where the patient's physician is already prescribing a psychotropic medication; or when you sense that the patient would be resistant to considering psychological intervention.

When calling a physician, begin by outlining your observations about the patient's behavior in the dental environment. Then emphasize that you believe that the patient's psychological status at this time appears to make him incapable of receiving dental treatment from any regular practitioner. While primary physicians are not experts in psychiatric assessment and treatment, most will have a reasonable understanding of the issues involved. Many will know appropriate professionals to whom they could refer the patient for specialized treatment.

You will sometimes find a patient who is receiving prescription medication such as an antidepressant, or an antianxiety drug, which appears to help her cope with the normal stresses of life, but who you feel is *still* too fearful to undergo regular dental care. Again it is appropriate for you to discuss this problem with the primary physician.

Ask the physician if she knows a mental health specialist whom the patient could work with in order to learn additional skills for coping more effectively in the dental environment.

Another problem you will occasionally face is the fearful dental patient who has not sought medical care for many years, and who you feel should see a physician before beginning dental treatment. Telling this patient to "find a doctor" will probably result in her simply disappearing. You are much more likely to succeed if you give her the name of a specific family practitioner who has a reputation for appropriate treatment. Once the patient agrees to go, it is important for you to telephone the physician to outline your concerns, and to alert him that he will have a terrified patient on his hands. If you are unfamiliar with such a physician, call your state or county medical association and ask for a family physician with a reputation for handling such patients.

Making a Referral to a Mental Health Specialist

When possible, a direct referral to a psychologist or psychiatrist is the best choice in cases where there are significant barriers to the patient's successfully completing care. Few dentists will have the name of a therapist handy for referral. What do you look for, and what do you say? In most communities there are psychologists and psychiatrists who specialize in the treatment of Anxiety Disorders such as specific phobias, Agoraphobia, Panic Disorder, or Generalized Anxiety Disorder. The therapeutic approaches which have been most successful in quickly resolving these problems are known as *Behavioral Therapy* and *Cognitive-Behavioral Therapy*. If you do not know an appropriate therapist, we recommend that you call your county or state psychological or psychiatric association. Either organization can refer you to professionals with the skills necessary to help your patient. In general, psychologists tend to be somewhat more familiar with the behavioral therapies, and less oriented to using psychotropic drugs. Psychiatrists are generally equipped to deal better with more disturbed patients and rely more frequently on various types of drug therapies. Again a telephone conversation about your patient will help you determine if he could benefit from psychological services.

If the patient is currently in therapy, it is appropriate to ask permission to speak with the therapist if you feel that he or she may have difficulty tolerating treatment. Again you must clearly state that you believe the patient's fears are so great that neither you, nor any other dentist you know, could successfully treat him or her at this point. If the current therapist is working with the patient about "family" or other personal issues, it is appropriate to ask some questions. Is he experienced in working with behavioral strategies to resolve phobias and anxiety disorders? Does he know of a colleague who could work with your patient on this specific issue.

Making a Referral to an Allergist

As we mentioned previously in the discussion of anesthetics and again regarding amalgam, there are some situations in which a referral to an allergist is appropriate. The patient who fears a medical catastrophe believes that the problem is a result of some dental procedure or chemical, not of fear. Making a referral to an allergist may be useful in helping reduce the patient's fears, but it requires careful planning. First, select the allergist yourself. Choose a well respected senior practitioner who understands that *how* information about test results and the consequences of the findings are presented is a large part of practice. Second, brief the allergist before the patient's appointment to increase the probability that a referral accomplishes your goals. Explain the purpose of your referral and your hypothesis for the cause of the patient's reaction. Even the best allergist will generally be less familiar with the safety issues regarding dental anesthetics than you are. Consequently, it would helpful to include a recent reference from the dental literature which discusses the extreme rarity of true allergic reactions. Third, explain that your goal is to rule out an allergic response. The way in which the allergist presents the findings is crucial. Imagine that he or she says something like, "I have tested you and you showed no reaction. Of course you could develop a reaction or sensitivity in the future although the chances are less than one-in-a-million. I would advise you to avoid this drug when possible to reduce any probability of an adverse reaction." Your patient will *always* conclude that he is the "One-in-a-million!!" Ask the allergist to state his findings to the patient in an authoritative non-equivocal manner. For example, he might say, "Susan, I am happy to report that the results of our tests reveal that your body showed absolutely no allergic responses to the dental materials. Many people find dental treatment pretty difficult. The reaction you describe is most consistent with one that is triggered by your thoughts and feelings— like crying—rather than one triggered by an outside chemical agent."

As we have mentioned previously, a referral to an allergist should be part of a larger strategy to "rule out" in the patient's mind that the trigger of her responses is based on outside phenomena rather than on her own anxieties. However, in some cases these patients are wedded to their beliefs and prove difficult to treat.

Using the expertise and services of other professionals is fundamental to dental practice. However, planning is essential in order to integrate a referral into a successful treatment plan, especially with the anxious or fearful patient.

QUESTIONS AND EXERCISES

1. We presented two conceptual models that relate one's thoughts to fears or emotional responses. Explain the differences between these two models. What are their similarities? Give an example which illustrates each of these two conceptualizations.

2. Identify a patient who has a specific fear of dentistry. Interview this patient to determine how his or her cognitive activity contributes to the apprehension he felt. Which of the two models applies? Determine ahead of time how you would present this information to the patient as an explanation for his response. Make a presentation to the patient and solicit his feedback to see if your explanation appeared reasonably accurate to him. Devise

and carry out a treatment plan for this patient's fear that is integrated within your dental treatment plan.

3. List the sequence of strategies you would use when a new patient told you that she could not allow you to use lidocaine with epinepherine because she was told by her previous dentist that she might be allergic.

4. Outline a hierarchy of steps for desensitizing a patient to radiographs. Describe the homework assignments you might give a patient.

5. List three questions that you could ask a patient fearful of injections which would help you assess the severity of the patient's fears.

6. What are three causes of adverse psychophysiological reactions to local anesthetic?

NINE

Periodontal Health

- Making Oral Hygiene a Priority
- Oral Hygiene Instruction
- Conservative Periodontal Therapy

MAKING ORAL HYGIENE A PRIORITY

While most of this book is addressed to helping the dental care team provide successful dental treatment experiences for fearful patients, the long-term prognosis for all patients is poor if they do not routinely practice a moderate level of oral self-care. That is why we have a special chapter on periodontal care in this textbook.

Many fearful patients are caught in an endless cycle of pain, emergencies, painful temporary treatment, and worry. Many adopt the attitude that their teeth and gums are like old "clunker" cars. Rather than do regular maintenance, and change the oil and the wipers, they just drive the old car into the ground and then junk it. To most health professionals, this attitude is illogical and it is tempting to try to motivate patients like this by stressing the benefits of treatment and better oral health. Surprisingly, this strategy often does not work.

Even the most fearful patients, are fully aware that effective dental treatment can bring great benefits. Nevertheless, they see many barriers in being able to endure the actual treatment. They know that *other* people can tolerate treatment; it is their own abilities they doubt. Consequently, they often resign themselves to something less than good health. It is easy to misread poor hygiene, inflamed gums, and broken-down teeth as "not caring." What is most interesting is that these patients are often great candidates for miracle makeovers in the hands of a capable dental hygienist or dentist. We spend a lot of effort planning how to make treatment easier and simpler for fearful patients. Since it is obvious that "regular dentistry" has not been successful in the past, the emphasis must be on gradually re-introducing the patient to dental care.

Professional tooth cleaning and conservative periodontal care are often the avenues we use to introduce fearful patients to all of the stimuli of dentistry. Because the procedures can be short, such as scaling and root planing a sextant or quadrant, we can make the "lesson" for the new patient easy enough so that it is not an overwhelming barrier to entering treatment.

Beginning treatment with periodontal health issues also gives us the opportunity to improve the patient's gingival health before doing any restorative dentistry or even extractions. This approach makes everything from the application of the rubber dam to post-operative complications easier and more predictable. No dentist likes to place a rubber dam if the gingiva bleeds profusely when touched. Similarly, the chances of post-operative problems may be increased after an extraction in a mouth with a lot of concurrent infection.

In most cases, having short weekly visits is the best management strategy. Dental hygienists need to be specifically instructed to adapt the treatment to the patient and not vice-versa. That is, the emphasis should be on patient learning and success.

One of the most common complaints of new patients in the Dental Fears Research Clinic regarding past treatment is, "They made me feel so guilty for having such bad teeth (gums)." It is very easy for a fearful patient who feels both guilt and embarrassment for "letting himself go" to perceive even innocent remarks as criticism. De Jongh (1993) found that only 15 percent of patients reported no anxiety about dental hygiene treatment. However, it is not uncommon for both hygienists and dentists to convey an attitude of judgment and disapproval. It is important for us to remember and convey to the patient that we are in a profession which treats illness, and not simply in the business of health maintenance for highly motivated patients with healthy teeth and gingiva.

Recall that every fearful patient needs a series of successful appointments in order to overcome fears and learn to be a good patient. You should emphasize learning and practicing coping skills as you introduce dental stimuli in a graded fashion. For example, the sonic scaler may be considered a surrogate for the high-speed drill. Thus, we will instruct the hygienist to "find a reason" to use it, knowing it will prepare the patient for much of what is to follow. Fear treatment is a team effort and the dentist must communicate a plan to the dental hygienist. If the patient is doing well during periodontal treatment, root tips can be removed during one of these appointments, taking the patient a further step toward health.

ORAL HYGIENE INSTRUCTION

We try to integrate targeted home care instruction into our initial cleaning appointments (Weinstein *et al.*, 1991). That is, when we scale and root plane the lower anterior teeth, we teach tooth brushing there. We find that it is sometimes difficult for our staff to confine their educational efforts solely to toothbrushing a small area when the mouth is such a mess. The principle behind our efforts is consistent with the fear treatment: graded exposure and consistent success in small steps. It took quite a while for the patient's dental problem to develop and it will take some time for it to be resolved. Emphasize to staff that their initial goal is to keep the patient coming back!

Some long-time avoiders have, without professional assistance, developed and adhered to an adequate regimen. These patients, albeit a minority, are consciously trying to compensate for a lack of professional supervision. They eagerly accept information that will help them enhance the effectiveness and efficiency of their regimens. Maintaining optimal oral health based on a concern for the consequences of neglect can be appropriate. On the other hand, the vast majority of such patients either do not maintain a daily regimen of oral self-care or they clean superficially or ineffectively. Many of these patients have disease-ravaged mouths that give new meaning to the "bombed-out" metaphor. Such mouths are difficult and painful to clean. One can imagine the downward spiral of avoidance of care, deterioration and decay, difficulty of self-care, and subsequent deterioration of health.

Competent health professionals in many disciplines are frequently stymied when they present preventive or therapeutic regimens either as prescriptions or proscriptions for patient behavior. Even when the prescription is easily within patients' power, e.g., taking a pill, many do not comply with professional advice. Researchers believe that 30 percent to 70 percent of all recommendations for home care, medication, diet, or exercise are not followed by patients. A 50 percent rate of noncompliance in self-reported frequency of brushing or flossing (or both) has emerged as the high watermark of success in primary preventive activities with normal dental patients. Standard approaches to oral hygiene instruction result in short-term gains but most patients relapse to old habits within months of any visit (Milgrom *et al.*, 1989; Weinstein *et al.*, 1989).

The next few pages specify basic behavioral principles necessary in plaque control. These are especially important in working with fearful patients.

Communication Is Critical

Be very cautious when you introduce plaque control programs. How you introduce patients to an oral self-care program may greatly influence their decision to agree to alter their present habits.

Many patients, even those with terrible hygiene, believe that they are already doing a pretty acceptable job of cleaning their teeth. Some patients may even feel slighted or coerced by comments suggesting that they are incompetent in oral self-care. You need to be careful when introducing plaque control because simply raising the topic may imply criticism of the patient's present habits.

The initial hygiene appointment may or may not be the best time to introduce plaque control techniques, even though that is customary. A non-individualized approach may jeopardize plaque control programs, especially with fearful, distrustful patients. To influence the patient's thinking and action, the dentist, hygienist, and assistant must be aware of her dental needs and goals. Sometimes, initial home care instruction is important because it helps give the patient a sense of control or enhances comfort. However, it is often assumed that when the patient understands the cause of the disease and the effectiveness of preventive health practice, her behavior will change. Research firmly indicates that information alone does not lead to altered behavior. By the time they reach the seventh grade, almost all children have heard that smoking is dangerous to their health, and yet, by this time, approximately 20 percent are already smoking. Old myths die hard.

Gold (1974) notes that many dentists who tell their patients about plaque control are often unaware that *how* they are relating to the patient is more important than *what* they are relating. The "how" of the doctor-patient interaction is the process of communication. The act of motivating a patient involves showing concern, listening, and providing information. Listening skills are critical, as is the expression of personal concern. Patients may judge concern by the amount of time the professional spends listening and discussing the patients' problems. Information has a secondary role in motivating patients.

Assess Readiness

At a given point, many people are not willing to consider altering their present self-care patterns, and some may never be ready. Dentist or hygienist pressure may result in a superficial acquiescence, and the patient may even attempt to try the new self-care behavior. However, the probability of creating long-term change is minimal.

It is useful to identify fearful patients who are likely or unlikely to respond to efforts to alter their self-care behavior. Patients who are likely to respond can be introduced to plaque control; you can discuss alternative procedures, frequent recall prophylaxes, and fluorides, for example, with those who are unlikely to respond to the plaque control approach.

There has been little dental research that attempts to identify those who are ready to alter self-care habits. However, there is some evidence that a history of an active role in maintaining health, e.g., exercise regimes, controlled diet, or elimination of smoking, is a positive predictor. The patient's stated intent to change when questioned is also useful. In all, when the patient perceives that he has a problem, and has a preventive orientation ("holistic" is a trendy term used to describe such health-consciousness) or a history of careful self-care, he is ready to alter sub-optimal patterns of dental cleaning. We find that fearful patients who have just made the crucial decision to seek dental care after a period of avoidance are often very good candidates for home care instruction.

Skill Level

Careful assessment of patient self-care practice is important. Although plaque control instruction often focuses on skill training, dentists and auxiliaries often do not systematically evaluate patient skills *before* instruction. This is a little more time-consuming, but the effort is invaluable when the instruction is being tailored to the patient's needs.

Knowledge of how the patient cleans her teeth at home can only come from observation of the patient's skills. We find that a patient will attempt to perform optimally, when asked to demonstrate skills, spending much time and effort to clean. As the patient attempts to avoid embarrassment, awkward and unfamiliar manipulations of instruments may become evident. When you assess skills, you should stress that you are interested in seeing his "at home" routine and that showing extraordinary effort in optimal cleansing is not useful.

The demonstration of routine "at home" self-care practices frequently discloses serious deficiencies. Often what is most striking is that the patient has no pattern or system for cleaning. Brushing appears almost random as the patient moves haphazardly from place to place. The lingual surfaces are the areas most commonly omitted during tooth brushing. Kleber and others (1981) showed that more than 80 percent of the children in a study failed to brush the lingual surfaces of the mandibular or maxillary teeth. Overall, 38 percent of the dental surfaces were not brushed. MacGreggor and Rugg-Gunn (1979) have similarly observed that the anterior labial surfaces were brushed most often and the lingual surfaces least often.

Findings for adults are no different. In 1946, Robinson found that tooth brushing was almost entirely confined to labial surfaces. More recently, Cumming and Löe (1973) found that labial surfaces had less plaque than lingual surfaces. Dexterity, even in adults, may be a factor. Kenney and others (1976) determined that manual dexterity of the preferred hand showed significant correlation with oral hygiene scores.

Observations of patient self-care are useful when you are deciding what to teach the patient. Subsequent use of disclosing tablets after cleaning serves to reinforce the idea that inefficient or ineffective cleaning of certain surfaces results in the accumulation of plaque. To improve any physical skill, you must provide feedback. Feedback about performance may come from a number of sources. Visual examination, disclosing solution, and self-inspection manuals can facilitate the feedback process (Baab & Weinstein, 1983). Patients must learn how to identify the problems in their own mouths.

Easily Attainable Goals

Once you have identified patient skill levels, then establish realistic and easily attainable goals or targets. We find that most professionals tend to go too far, too fast. The behavioral approach must proceed slowly, step by step, with considerable encouragement for the accomplishment of each step.

With patients whose skill levels are very low, or for whom cleaning is difficult because of broken-down teeth, overhangs, and advanced periodontitis, we focus on the thorough cleaning of only a few teeth, usually the anterior teeth that are to be repaired, or have just received curettage. On subsequent appointments, we give patients detailed feedback and encouragement. As the patient makes progress, we can focus on additional teeth. This incremental approach works well with patients who have regular but ineffective home care habits. As a general rule, *no patient should be given more than one cleaning aid until the previous one is mastered.* In our opinion, until the patient demonstrates consistent effective use of the tooth-brush it is almost counterproductive to introduce toothpicks, perio aids, or proxibrushes. We have found patients are less resistant to mastering a current activity such as brushing than adopting a new one. Because it is so difficult to use well, dental floss should be reserved for the "advanced" patient or the rare person who actually likes to floss.

We recommend disclosing the fearful patient's teeth at every visit, not to criticize but to help him see plaque and evaluate his progress. This allows us to function as coaches. We watch our "athletes" perform and then give feedback designed to improve their skills. Praise and encouragement of the patient's efforts are crucial.

We also recommend brushing without toothpaste. This allows patients to see the teeth and evaluate their gums. Toothpaste makes it difficult to see bleeding resulting from unresolved gingivitis.

Facilitate Transfer of New Skills

Though patients may want to alter their behaviors, old habits often interfere. As a general principle, learning to make new responses to familiar situations produces "negative transfer"; that is, the intrusion of old automatic habits into new behaviors. For instance, once a patient is home, her old way of brushing may replace the new techniques learned at your office. To facilitate transfer of this skill, we try to help patients make their oral care a self-conscious activity. Looking into a well-lighted mirror when cleaning may help the patient because patients are taught new skills in the office using a mirror. Reminders are useful, such as monitoring charts and notes placed on mirrors or where oral self-care occurs. A copy of a chart we find useful is found in Figure 9-1. These charts are also useful in helping to establish realistic goals and objectives and they provide considerable feedback. All of these instructions are designed to help the patients perceive the differences between their old habits and the new skills they have learned. Just as important, they tend to help the patient remember to substitute the new habit for the old.

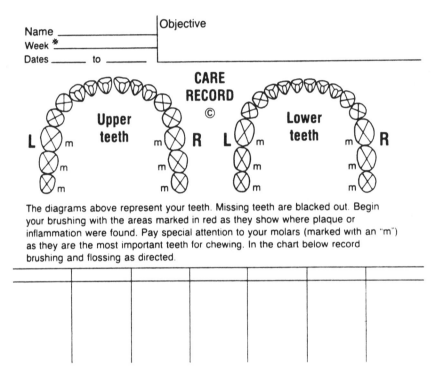

Name _____

Week * _____

Dates _____ to _____

Objective

CARE RECORD ©

Upper teeth

Lower teeth

L m   m R   L m   m R

The diagrams above represent your teeth. Missing teeth are blacked out. Begin your brushing with the areas marked in red as they show where plaque or inflammation were found. Pay special attention to your molars (marked with an "m") as they are the most important teeth for chewing. In the chart below record brushing and flossing as directed.

Compliance versus Cooperation

A capable clinician will evaluate every appointment. Was the fear-reduction goal met? Was the periodontal treatment goal met? Was the self-care goal met? One very important step is to debrief the patient. It doesn't take long but the information is essential. With regard to the oral hygiene instruction, it might go something like this:

Hygienist: Well, today I introduced you to a new way to use your toothbrush on your lower front teeth. Do you have any questions about doing this at home?

Patient: No, I don't think so.

Hygienist: Good. Does this seem like something you will actually be able to fit into your schedule?

It is easiest for the overwhelmed patient to agree to cooperate in your presence without actually feeling that he is able to carry out your recommendations. If you ask directly, you may find this out. If that is the case, your lesson plan included too much. Try to take smaller steps and reduce what you are asking the patient to accomplish. Based on our experience, this will produce more success.

Weinstein, Getz, and Milgrom (1991) describe the steps of this approach in detail in their handbook *Oral Self Care: Strategies for Preventive Dentistry*. Over the last few years considerable data have been collected that point to the effectiveness of this approach.

Finances

When patients need multiple scaling and root planing visits there is often ample opportunity for many self-care lessons and practice of fear reduction strategies that don't take a lot of extra time. This is particularly true because we advocate very small steps. Remember, it often takes many repetitions of the same lesson before patients catch on. Some of our patients do not show changes until after several maintenance visits. Thus, the key is to keep the patient coming back so that you can re-deliver the message and reinforce any progress. In this case, the fee for the periodontal procedures may be adequate and the instructional time can be included without extra charge. Often dentists feel that the overall rewards associated with the patient's rehabilitation are more than enough to compensate for a little extra up-front time. They view it as a cost of doing business similar to the cost of an extra appointment for redoing a bridge or crown impression that was not quite good enough.

On the other hand, if the patient's oral hygiene skills are very poor, or the dental hygienist is primarily providing a "little bit of hygiene" in the context of desensitization and fear management, it is appropriate that the patient be charged a fee for these additional visits on a time basis. Other practices are most comfortable quoting an up-front fee, for example $100-$300, which is later refunded or applied to the cost of other procedures if the patient follows through with the overall treatment plan. We explain the importance of these services by emphasizing that teaching good home care skills and helping a patient learn to tolerate treatment comfortably are the two most important services that we provide. We find that few patients object to approaching their health from a perspective of "wellness" even though their insurance company pays only for "repairs." Different strategies work for different patients and the best approach is to be flexible

CONSERVATIVE PERIODONTAL THERAPY

This is clearly the decade of conservative approaches to periodontal therapy. Even when open flap procedures may be contemplated in the future, initial therapy almost always includes closed scaling and root planing. There is considerable evidence for its success (see, for example, Egelberg, 1992). Because many patients have heard that periodontal therapy is painful and expensive, you need to explain what you are proposing, and we strongly suggest avoiding periodontal surgery in any initial plan.

Often, at chairside, our clinical staff in the Dental Fears Research Clinic describe the treatment as similar to removing a bad splinter. Left to itself, the splinter can create inflammation, swelling, and even pus. Removing the splinter and washing out the cut allow the body to heal. Periodontal treatment is roughly the same except that the architecture of the mouth requires different instruments and strategy. This type of presentation demystifies the problem and reduces worry. This is not the time for selling the patient on the treatment plan; the dentist should have taken that step initially. At this point, we are trying only to explain the nature of the problem and the disease, using situations the patient can easily understand. For example, we might say, "Periodontal disease is somewhat like diabetes. We know how to control it through regular care and maintenance, but we do not know how to cure it. And, just like with diabetes 90 percent of the success is determined by what you do every day to keep yourself healthy."

Patients may need mucogingival procedures or resective surgery at some point. Crown lengthening may be important in final rehabilitation. Nevertheless, these procedures need to be postponed until the patient has adequate coping skills.

Pain Control

There should be absolutely no periodontal treatment of fearful patients without anesthetics and analgesics. These issues are discussed in detail in Chapter 7. Pain is often magnified in fearful patients, who anticipate the worst. Thus, it is the clinician's responsibility to use pain control methods effectively. This is not the time to ask the patient whether or not he would prefer local anesthetic. Decisions about pain control should be made as part of the overall treatment plan. Our advice is to err on the side of too much rather than too little pain control.

Probing hurts! From the patient's view, how can he tolerate treatment if the exam is so terrible? We do not probe obvious periodontal defects at the initial exam. Overwhelming or hurting the patient in the name of thoroughness will too often result in his failing to proceed with treatment. You can obtain accurate probings as the patient is anesthetized for initial periodontal therapy. Periapical radiographs or even vertical bite-wing films provide key information. Such an approach maximizes patient comfort and still allows adequate documentation. We tend to use local anesthetic liberally. Since the area to be treated at each appointment is small, the time burden in using anesthetics is relatively minor and allows the patient to learn about injections and experience pain-free care. This strategy is worth considering even when state law does not allow the dental hygienist to administer local anesthetic and the dentist must be involved.

As with all treatment, getting patient feedback on comfort is essential. Initially, a single stroke with a curette should be followed with a question to the patient about pain. Any pain responses should be dealt with. Remember, expressing concern and pain-free treatment is part of the overall fear management process. If you are late or in a hurry because of your schedule, it is better to shorten the care and make another appointment rather than hurrying and hurting the patient. High quality technique and thoroughness are always essential and your pain control strategies allow this.

When the gingival and periodontal disease situation warrants it, we often employ chlorhexidine gluconate rinses or antibiotics before actually beginning conservative periodontal treatment. The rationale for this strategy is to reduce the amount of bleeding and discomfort associated with treatment. If you properly explain this, the patient sees it as reducing any discomfort associated with initial treatment, again a barrier-lowering step. It is a good idea to have a supply of chlorhexidine on hand in the office and let the patient try it for "taste." If he rejects the taste in the office, it is unlikely he will follow through. We always ask directly, "Does this seem like something you can do?" or "Will you do this?" If he rejects it, don't cajole the patient into accepting the drug; it won't work. In that case, use antibiotics if appropriate or even an over-the-counter rinse if you think it will help.

One special case is the patient with a substance abuse history, particularly those who are members of Alcoholics Anonymous. These patients may reject the alcohol-based chlorhexidine rinse available. This is also true for patients who find the alcohol-based rinse painful. In order to overcome this problem, we developed an alternative rinse that you may be able to have prepared in your community pharmacy:

> 0.12% chlorhexidine rinse from a 20% aqueous chlorhexidine solution (Spectradyne-G™, Lonza) with 10% glycerin, peppermint oil (2 drops/960 ml), blue color (2 drops/960 ml), and water (Milgrom *et al.*, 1992).

As discussed in Chapter 7, a loading dose of a non-steroidal anti-inflammatory medication may be appropriate before scaling and root planing. Similarly, a specific strategy for post-operative pain management is important. This might range from warm water rinses or using chlorhexidine to using aspirin, acetaminophen, ibuprofen, or prescription pain medications. Most patients can tell you what works for them and it is perilous to ignore what they say. Refer to Chapter 7 for more information on what medications to employ.

Transferring from the Dental Hygienist to the Dentist

Once the patient has made progress in the periodontal arena we will often schedule a brief reassessment visit before proceeding with restorative treatment. This allows us to clarify the goals, treatment time, and finances. It also allows us to reassess whether or not additional fear reduction strategies are needed.

If the dental hygienist has already given the patient an injection, we may continue that pattern by having the hygienist give the injection for the restorative treatment or surgery and then assist the dentist in the first new procedure. Patients are often reassured by this continuity. If the dentist has previously given the injections as part of the periodontal treatment, this may not be necessary. Nevertheless, the concept of trying to provide continuity between providers is important.

Sometimes there is a *purposeful* conversation between the dentist and the dental hygienist in front of the patient.

Dentist: Mary [the hygienist], are there any special recommendations you have for me in working with Mr. Garcia?

Mary: Yes, Mr. Garcia's back gets tired during treatment. We have found that this pillow and letting him stand every 20 minutes or so really helps.

Dentist: Okay, anything else?

Mary: Yes. Mr. Garcia has really learned some very good breathing skills. After you place the topical anesthetic, you need to give him a little while to get calmed down before the injection. He will signal you with his hand when he is ready for you to proceed. Structuring time during the injection is also very helpful.

Patients find this type of conversation reassuring. That way, everyone in the practice knows the "ground rules"—the strategies that have been developed to maximize the patient's psychological and physical comfort. In this situation it would be useful for the dentist to ask the patient if there was anything else he should know which would make it easier for the patient.

Recall Frequency

After the patient completes the initial course of periodontal therapy, he should be placed on what we call a "short leash." That is, the initial recall should be in about one month, followed by two months, and so on until an optimal recall period is established. No patient who began treatment fearful and neglectful should be placed on even a three-month recall interval. We are building new habits and they are very difficult to establish. In other words, we are not concerned that the patient's oral health will have deteriorated in a single month and need our care. Instead we recognize that the patient needs continuing reminders and reinforcement both in coming to the dentist and in performing her newly acquired habits. These initial sessions may be quite short and focus on oral hygiene checks, or on therapy for two or three specific periodontically compromised teeth. The practice needs to use all of its "tricks" to get this patient on to the recall system. Reminder phone calls, postcards, birthday cards, and whatever else is available should be used. This step is absolutely critical to the success of your efforts.

What about referrals to periodontists?

As we discussed in Chapter 8, referrals are effective only when there is a relationship between the referring dentist and the patient. Thus, attempts to refer patients during the initial phase of treatment will most often be unsuccessful. Patients will not go. After all, they just barely had enough courage to come to you! It is important to keep a long-term perspective on the problem. If the patient does not follow through on the referral, or has a bad experience with the specialist, it is highly likely he will not return to your practice out of guilt or embarrassment. Ideally, a patient should finish the initial course of scaling and root planing and be on periodontal maintenance through several cycles *before* any referral. Moreover, you need to have excellent written and oral consultation with the periodontist before making a referral to be sure that he has, and is willing to use, the patient management skills you have developed. Otherwise, even an examination visit with painful probing can undo all of your good efforts.

SUMMARY

In this chapter we have discussed periodontal care for the fearful patient. The majority of fearful patients lack good home care skills, and periodontal problems are common. Oral hygiene instruction and conservative periodontal care are frequently a good introduction for the fearful patient to the dental environment. They allow for instruction, graduated exposure, and can serve to prepare the patient for restorative procedures. When the hygienist is the first member of the team to work with a fearful patient, he or she should be given the flexibility to work with the patient slowly. A working relationship with the referring dentist and close communication about fear reduction strategies is critical to "transfer" the patient to the care of another professional.

QUESTIONS AND EXERCISES

1. How can oral hygiene instruction and initial periodontal care enhance fear reduction?

2. Consider a "theoretical" 40-year-old patient with generalized 6-8 mm periodontal pockets, early furcation involvements in the molars, extensive gingivitis and poor oral hygiene. Create a step-wise model treatment plan for periodontal care.

3. List the steps you would use in pain control for conservative periodontal treatments.

4. Describe some of the common reasons why most efforts at changing oral hygiene fail to alter the patients home care habits.

TEN

Treating Fearful Children

- Creating a Safe Environment
- Assessment Procedures
- Preventive Steps Worth Taking
- Effective Management in the Operatory
- Pharmacological Management Techniques

Some dental health professionals are reluctant to treat children because they may be difficult to manage. Lack of training and experience with children and the attitude that treating children is not rewarding may exacerbate the problem. Students and clinicians not experienced in treating children often are not confident of their ability. This itself may contribute to difficulties (Weinstein *et al.*, 1981).

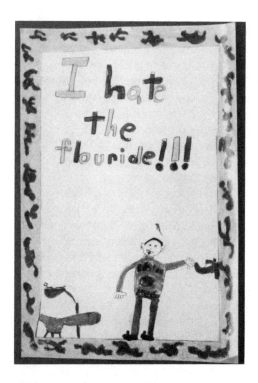

Although strategies delineated in the previous chapters can be effective for patients of all ages, we have added this chapter to discuss special considerations for children because the goals for treating this age group differ from the general treatment goals for adults. Studies by experts in the field of childhood and pain, such as Milgrom *et al.* (1988); Forgione and Clark (1974); Kleinknecht *et al.* (1973); Lautch (1971); and Shoben and Borland (1954), show that most people feel that their dental fears began in childhood. Creating positive attitudes toward dental care in children is an effective strategy to shape positive attitudes toward dentistry in adults, and as such is a major goal of all treatment for children. Altering phobias is much more difficult and expensive. Early dental experiences should occur with a minimum of physical and psychological trauma.

Clinicians as far back as the turn of the century were concerned about the child's fear of dentistry. In 1895, McElroy noted: "Although the operative dentistry may be perfect, the appointment is a failure if the child departs in tears." Just as standard restorative, endodontic, and orthodontic techniques have been modified to treat deciduous dentition, the need to alter patient management has also been recognized. In fact, dental practitioners have long realized that the child's behavior is the most important factor affecting actual treatment. Without patient cooperation, all dental procedures become difficult. Moreover, we now realize that today's treatment of the child is useful in laying a foundation for his future acceptance of dental treatment. The need for effective, humane behavior management of children is obvious.

This chapter on treating children could easily have been expanded into a book. We wrote it to be of practical use to students and clinicians treating children and it stems from our research and clinical experience. We begin by discussing the need for creating a safe environment for children and then discuss, in detail, a variety of topics: child and parent assessment procedures; procedures for preventive management of problems, including introducing the child to the office; enhancing a sense of control and coping; controversy about parents in the operatory; and effective management in the operatory. Toward the end of the chapter we include the following topics: general principles, i.e., what to do and what not to do when interacting with children; the appropriate role of the assistant; special consideration for older children and teenagers; and a discussion of aversive techniques and alternatives. The use of pharmacologic adjuncts for children follows. We also refer the reader to our discussions of nitrous oxide and premedication in Chapter 7 and to texts and articles in child management, for example, the Ripa and Barenie (1979) text and the Weinstein and Nathan (1988) article. Recently, Rayman (1994) has reviewed the contemporary pediatric literature and recommends dental and non-dental books useful in managing pediatric dental patients.

THE GOAL: CREATING A SAFE PSYCHOLOGICAL ENVIRONMENT

Towards the aim of providing humane treatment, our goal is to create an accepting, "safe" child-oriented environment, a place for the child to explore and learn. We simply want the child to learn that the dental office is not scary and that he has the opportunity to cope with dental procedures. In doing so we recognize that children and adults are different and that developmental factors are at work. For example, young children have difficulty separating from their parents in a strange environment, and that while adults tend not to exhibit their fears, children have far fewer inhibitions.

When a child is afraid, it is very helpful to provide acknowl-edgment of her subjective experience. Statements that elicit child feelings let her know that we care enough to ask. After the child has expressed her feelings, we thank her for sharing them and express understanding and empathy. We try to avoid reassuring the child prematurely ("Everything will be okay").

Most children seen in the dental office are cooperative and allow the staff to function effectively and efficiently. As a result of long-term water fluoridation, topical fluoride applications and sealants, and the widespread use of fluoridated dentifrices, children are less likely to need frequent restorative care. Without traumatic restorative care, children are not as likely to misbehave. Of the minority who do misbehave, few present problems that are serious enough to disrupt treatment. Most misbehavior, such as whining or crying, is merely irritating. Although the practitioner needs patience and the ability to "wait it out," the child eventually comes to realize that his behavior will not produce its intended result and that other behaviors are more productive. Other misbehaviors, such as passive refusal to "open wide" or shouts of "I won't" or "I don't want to," or hyperactivity—inability to sit still for more than a minute or so—can disrupt efficient treatment. The child who throws a tantrum—screams and flails legs and arms—not only disrupts treatment but endangers his own and the staff's well-being. Although there are procedures to manage disruptive and dangerous child behavior, measures you take to prevent such extreme behavior from emerging from existing anxiety or fear are well worth the effort.

Early in this chapter we focus on some techniques that you can use when working with children to *prevent* problems from developing or becoming unmanageable. Later in this chapter we will discuss management of these problems.

Survey of Child Management Problems

Weinstein *et al.* (1981) reported the results of surveying 145 Washington State general practitioners. An average of one-third of all patients seen per week (21/60) were children. Of that number, 6.5 percent presented difficulties. Fifteen percent of the practitioners reported that 20 percent or more of their child patients are problematic. Infants and toddlers were the most difficult age group to manage. Rates of successful treatment for problem categories were as follows: inability to communicate (29 percent), lack of cooperation (50 percent), "out-of-control behavior" (61 percent), and fear and anxiety (75 percent).

Techniques used to manage difficult children ranged from hand-over-mouth, mouth props, premedication with nitrous oxide and diazepam (Valium®), to praise, desensitization, and careful explanation. No one technique was used by general practitioners significantly more often than other techniques or was more successful than any other. Pharmacological approaches were used in 26 percent of the difficult cases that were reported. These approaches were reported to be no more successful than non-drug approaches.

ASSESSMENT PROCEDURES

Questionnaires

Before discussing prevention, it is necessary to talk about assessment. Assessment should take place as early as possible, and information about parent and child is worth gathering. The parent in the reception room is often a source of information that can help you better manage the child. Exactly what information should be sought is a function of your individual practice. However, we believe that information that will help establish rapport and attune staff to possible behavior problems is extremely valuable. The following questions may be helpful:

1. Does the child have any pets, hobbies, special interests, or recent accomplishments?

   Yes   No

   If "yes," please list or give kind of pet and names.

2. Does the child have a nickname he enjoys?

   Yes   No

   If "yes," what is it?

3. Name of school, grade.

4. Other children in family?

   Yes   No

   Please give name, age, and sex of each.

5. Has the child had any unpleasant contact with physicians or dentists?

   Yes   No

   If "yes," please describe.

6. How do you think your child will react to dental treatment?

   Good   Fair   Poor   Don't know

   Please comment.

7. How fearful are you of having your dental work done?

   Not at all   A little fearful   Somewhat fearful   Very fearful

8. How would you rate your own anxiety or nervousness at this moment?

   Good   Fair   Poor   Don't know

9. Has your child had behavior or learning problems at school?

   Yes   No

   Please describe problems.

10. Does your child express concern about aspects of his teeth or mouth, such as a chipped or crooked tooth, decayed tooth, gum boil, etc.?

Yes   No

If "yes," please specify.

Studies attempting to identify factors influencing children's behavior in the dental office, summarized in a scholarly review by G.Z. Wright in 1975, have pinpointed three major variables. First, the pleasantness or unpleasantness of any previous medical experiences will affect a child's behavior during his first dental visit (Martin *et al.*, 1977). The similarity between dentist and physician is immediately obvious. Both are called doctor, wear white coats, and employ receptionists and auxiliaries who dress similarly. Fear, especially in children, is often generalized from one situation to another similar one (Bedi *et al.*, 1992). Second, in many studies (Johnson & Baldwin, 1968 and 1969; Wright & Alpern, 1971; Bailey *et al.*, 1973), maternal anxiety was found to be related to children's behavioral problems. Very anxious mothers have been found to exert a negative influence on children of all ages. Finally, the child's awareness of a dental problem also creates apprehension. This may manifest itself as uncooperative behavior in the dental chair (Wright *et al.*, 1973). Remember the anecdote about Joan in Chapter 1?

Not all problems in managing children are fear-related. Some children, even at a young age, chronically exhibit disruptive behaviors. At one extreme is the *hyperactive* child, who seems to have no control over his behavior. The clinical condition is characterized by excessive and unpredictable behaviors, unawareness of consequences, inability to focus on and concentrate on a task, and poor performance in school. Though not hyperactive, some children with little internal or external control of their impulses appear to mimic hyperactive behavior. Both actual and pseudo hyperactive children usually have had maladaptive patterns of attention with parents and demonstrate noncompliant behavior with other adults.

The following questionnaire, adapted from the work of Forehand and McMahon (1981), who provide therapy for children and their parents, provides information that can be used to help structure a brief discussion with parents. The behaviors receiving the top three ranks are likely to manifest themselves in the operatory.

Parent Behavior Checklist

Check the behaviors below that represent problem areas with your child. Then rank-order the behaviors you checked from the most frequent to the least frequent.

_____ 1. Whines

_____ 2. Is physically negative (attacks another person)

_____ 3. Is destructive (destroys, damages, or attempts to damage objects)

_____ 4. Uses smart talk (teases, makes fun of, or embarrasses others)

_____ 5. Is noncompliant (does not do what he or she is told to do)

_____ 6. Ignores (fails to answer)

_____ 7. Yells or screams

_____ 8. Demands attention

_____ 9. Has temper tantrums

A few other factors associated with child fear and its manifestations in the dental office are worth mentioning. Age of the child has been often associated with fear. Younger children generally show greater fear and less cooperation. Children under age 3 present the greatest difficulty, because communication between child and practitioner is difficult.

Socioeconomic class and gender are also factors. Low socioeconomic (poor) children are apt to be more frightened than their more affluent playmates (Hawley *et al.*, 1974; Wright, 1980). Moreover, boys show less fear than girls, a cultural or biological phenomenon.

The Preappointment Letter

We have noted that anxious mothers tend to have uncooperative children. Interestingly, researchers have found that when anxious mothers try to reduce their children's anxieties, they paradoxically increase anxiety. Apparently many mothers (and fathers) do not know how to prepare their children for dental visits. One practical approach to this problem involves sending a preappointment letter to parents of new child patients. In a study published in 1973, Wright, Alpern, and Leake report success with a letter that read like this:

Dear Mrs. _____:

I am writing you because I am pleased with the interest you are showing in your child's dental health by making an appointment for a dental examination. Children who have their first dental appointment when they are young are likely to have a favorable outlook toward dental care throughout life.

At our first appointment we will examine your child's teeth and gums, and take any necessary X-rays. For most children this proves to be an interesting and even pleasant occasion. All of the people on our staff enjoy children and know how to work with them.

Parents play a most important role in getting children started with a good attitude toward dental care, and your cooperation is much appreciated. One of the useful things that you can do is to be completely natural and easygoing when you tell your child about his appointment. This approach will enable him to view his appointment primarily as an opportunity to meet some new people who are interested in him and want to help him to stay healthy.

Good general health depends in large part upon the development of good habits, such as sensible eating and sleeping routines, exercise, recreation, and the like. Dental health also depends upon good habits, including proper tooth-brushing, regular visits for dental care, and avoidance of excessive sweets. We will have a chance to discuss these points further during your child's appointment.

Best wishes, and I look forward to seeing you.

You may want to send a short questionnaire, similar to the 10-item version given earlier, which asks for information on the child's interests, etc., with the letter.

Observation Checklists

In addition to questionnaires, your own observations are very valuable. Lists of behaviors to watch out for are helpful in collecting information. At times, especially when the child has had a history of difficulty receiving dental treatment, we ask the parent to direct the child in a structured activity and we observe the parent guiding the child. For example, "Mom, would you help Susie put this puzzle together?" or "After you watch me demonstrate, could you show Susie how to brush her teeth?" In the latter example, we ask an auxiliary to provide not only instruction, but also an assessment of how the mother functions. Occasionally a parent will be reluctant to interact with his child while being observed. Assure the parent that you understand, but that you want to see how the child interacts in this stressful, atypical dental setting.

We carefully observe parent and child not only in the waiting and treatment rooms but also during subsequent pre-visit activities and prophylaxis. Assessment is continuous. Chart notes always mention child and parent behavior and serve as a guide to future management. For example, the notation that the child cried during prophylaxis and asked repeatedly whether she would receive a "shot" is extremely helpful in developing an approach to the child for restorative treatment. Not knowing this information would be disastrous.

The following checklist may be part of a comprehensive assessment:

Brief Checklist for Waiting Room

1. Is child upset, neutral, unhappy?

2. Does child leave sight of parent (to explore, play, etc.)?

3 Does parent scold, threaten, or otherwise coerce child?

4. Does parent ignore or pay minimal attention to child, even when child is upset?

PREVENTIVE STEPS
WORTH TAKING FOR EVERY CHILD

Rapport and good communication go a long way to help the child feel comfortable in the dental environment. Careful introduction of the child to the dental environment, to enhance the child's sense of control and ability to cope will also help to reduce fear and promote the success of almost all children in tolerating dental treatment. At times this is best accomplished in a brief pre-treatment appointment.

Establish Rapport and Communicate Effectively

Establishing rapport, one of the foremost objectives when treating children, is not a "technique" that is applied for a few minutes at the beginning of each appointment. Rather, it is recognizing each child as a unique person. If you do not have rapport with the child, nothing else counts!

Rapport building phrases can be helpful, particularly with younger children, especially if they are humorous, such as, "Did you remember to bring your teeth today?" Older children's clothes, particularly the "billboard" tee-shirts, may give you clues to their interests. Taking a little time to learn about the child (including nickname, pets, hobbies, etc.) tells the child that he is cared for. On the other hand, your own unique way of responding to adults with whom you are comfortable is also the appropriate way to respond to children in establishing and maintaining rapport. The difference is that you use simpler concepts and vocabulary with children— without talking down to them. You should talk to children at their level of comprehension. That means avoiding baby talk: use words that have meaning for the patient. Developing of your own word substitutes for foreign (to children) dental terminology can be useful; for example, rubber dam becomes *rubber raincoat*; cotton roll becomes a *tooth pillow*; and a saliva ejector becomes a *thirsty straw*. Avoiding scary words such as drill, shot, pain, and using lay terms ("this will feel like a little pinch") will make difficult procedures more acceptable. Practice this as if it were a second language. Everyone in an office should try to use the same terminology.

There are many ways to break the ice with children. Questions about their clothing, activities, and pets are commonly used. Sometimes it is helpful to play with a child, especially one who is upset or apprehensive. A ball, balloons, dolls, and games, are all useful props in establishing human contact. Whatever the tactic for initiating a conversation, you should plan to use open-ended questions that cannot be responded to with a simple "yes" or "no." For example, do not ask whether the child has a pet—ask him to tell you all about his pets.

Nonverbal communication is also important in establishing rapport. Touching or patting a child's shoulder communicates warmth; smiles convey approval and acceptance. Eye contact is important—when talking to children place yourself at the child's eye level. There is probably some truth in the clinical lore which states that children who avoid eye contact are not ready to cooperate fully. One very common mistake involves assuming that all children of a particular chronological age think and feel the same. Though developmental trends permit some generalizations among children of the same chronological age, there is considerable variation in their social and mental development.

We believe, from our experience, that the behavior of the dentist and staff in the waiting room will set the tone for the initial and subsequent visits. The following sequence of rapport-building behaviors is recommended for preschool children:

1. Greet child and parent, child first, in the waiting room shortly after their arrival. Talk to the child for a short time. The "patter" will vary according to inclination and experience. We like to find a way to compliment the child, e.g., "I like your purple dinosaur shoes; they are neat!" Encourage a friendly dialogue, e.g., "Mom just got them for me." All sorts of interactions about clothing and movies are now possible, and about pets and animals, e.g., "Tell me about your pets." or "What animals do you like?" Sesame Street and holidays and birthdays are other ice breakers. When children are timid and do not respond, do not give up. Tell a brief story about something, e.g., "We have a dog named Josh. He is white with a curly tail and he likes children. This is his picture. Would you like to play with him?"

2. Introduce the child to toys. Tell him you will come back

soon and show him some other "neat stuff." Play with him for a minute.

3. Return and structure a choice for the child. While you take his hand, say "Now would you like to play with my special chair, or hold my special light (or brush or mirror)?"

4. If the child is very tentative, invite the parent to come in with you: "Mom, would you like to play with us too?" Most times, avoiding the trauma of separating the child from his parent is warranted. Moreover, parents can be very helpful if they are properly oriented to the role they will play. On the other hand, whether or not to allow the parent in the operatory is somewhat controversial.

5. Structure additional chores for the child: "Would you like to climb into the chair from this side (right side) or from here (left side)?"

6. Introduce everything. The "tell-show-do" approach, popularized by Addelston (1959), is extremely useful during initial appointments and in introducing complete-ly new procedures during subsequent appointments. The approach is very simple. First *tell* the child about each new procedure and what is going to be done in it. The initial oral exam may proceed as follows: "We are going to count your teeth with our tooth counter." *Show* the child the instruments and describe any sensation that he might feel in positive or neutral terms. "This (mirror) is my counter. I will gently touch each tooth as I count." If the child is at all tentative, demonstrate: "Let's count your fingers with the counter." Similarly, the child's fingernail may be "cleaned" to introduce the sight, sound, and vi-bration of the handpiece before prophylaxis. "Now, did you bring your teeth today?" At this point, do what you said you would do: "I see you have lots of pretty teeth. Let's count ..." In using this approach, be especially care-ful to use language and concepts that the child can under-stand.

7. Use lots of praise for any and all child cooperation.

Always complete the visit on a positive note. Help the child feel a sense of accomplishment. Point out that he did a good job and thank him.

8. Give children a small gift after treatment. The gift is provided *regardless* of their behavior. Though the behavioral literature indicates that such reinforcement should be provided contingent on appropriate behavior, it is our impression that the gift serves a useful function—it is a signal of accepting the child himself. Shapiro (1967) has suggested the possibility that a gift before the appointment may be more meaningful and helpful than a gift provided after the visit, and he has reported favorable responses of children to his pre-operative gift. We think Dr. Shapiro has a good idea.

9. Another good idea may be the "contingent" use of stories played through headphones. Nash *et al.* (1984) found that when story tapes were interrupted following uncooperative behavior and resumed when the child cooperated, fear-related behaviors were lower and cooperation was higher than in distraction (non-contingent use of story tapes) and control conditions.

Careful Introduction of the Child to the Dental Office

As discussed in Chapter 2, the genesis of much fear-related behavior in the dental office is poor early exposure to dentistry. Such harmful initiation may be *direct*, a result of stressful dental treatment, or it may be *indirect*, a result of frightening comments and anxiety of other children and adults (Milgrom *et al.*, 1994).

Mismanagement may exacerbate existing developmental problems. For example, separation of a protesting three-year-old from his mother and not allowing him to have control over any events are both management techniques that *enhance* fear and related behavior.

Much has been written about introducing children to dental treatment, usually emphasizing reassurance and explanation. These techniques have limited utility, especially with highly anxious children (Howitt & Stricker, 1977).

Pre-exposing children to a pleasant, low-stress dental experience was first reported in the early 1960s. Rosengarten (1961) brought children in for a pre-visit to introduce them to the office; he provided treatment during subsequent appointments. He found that children from 3 to 4.5 years old benefited, while those 5 to 5.5 years old did not. A few years later Laufer *et al.* (1964) used a similar technique with 6- to 7-year-old girls and found that the pre-visit significantly reduced fear.

Machen and Johnson (1974) compared two types of pre-visit intervention to a control condition. Preschool children with carious lesions were assigned to a control, desensitization, or modeling condition. After assignment to treatment groups, the experimental groups received the appropriate intervention one week prior to two restorative appointments. In the desensitization condition, procedures producing the least anxiety were presented first, followed by procedures that evoke more and more anxiety. The items related to these procedures and their order of presentation, from least to most "anxiety evoking," were as follows:

1. Prophylaxis contra-angle and pumice
2. Mirror and explorer
3. Rubber dam clamp
4. Rubber dam
5. Cavity liner
6. X-ray film
7. Handpiece
8. Anesthetic syringe
9. Dental operatory:
   a. Chair
   b. Light
   c. Water and air syringes
   d. Handpiece

The researchers noted that because the operatory itself is a high-anxiety stimulus, the intervention was held in an ordinary room until near the end of the session.

The modeling condition consisted of viewing an 11-minute videotape of a child showing positive behavior during dental treatment and being reinforced by the dentist. Results of this study indicated that both experimental groups had similar positive behavior during subsequent restorative treatment.

Overall, we believe that the evidence still supports the use of pre-visits for high-risk children who, because of existing caries or caries susceptibility, are likely to face stressful dental procedures. Those children who do not have caries or have a low caries susceptibility probably do not need such preparation, because dentistry for these children is not likely to be traumatic (Sawtell *et al.*, 1974; Rouleau *et al.*, 1981).

For children with no previous dental experience, we recommend that those between ages 3 and 5 be carefully introduced to the dental environment, but without a pre-visit. There may be good reason for careful introduction to the dental environment even earlier for high-risk children.

The comforting behaviors of the dentist and the staff are critical. For example, Sawtell and colleagues (1974) found a friendly assistant to be as effective as desensitization and other treatments. Clearly, accomplishing dental procedures is secondary. Allowing the child to play while waiting in the dental office is a widely accepted pedodontic practice. A few pieces of child-size furniture and toys are all that are necessary. Play communicates to the child that the people who work here are child oriented.

Modeling may be especially useful. The modeling management strategy used by Machen and Johnson (1974) deserves elaboration because it may be implemented in conjunction with other management approaches. Allowing the child to observe another patient undergoing treatment is based on the assumption that information about what to expect and how to behave contributes to reducing fear and subsequent behavior problems.

The most critical factor determining the effectiveness of the modeling procedure is that the person perceives the model as similar to himself. In other words, a 7-year-old boy watching a 13-year-old girl would not help the boy very much. It may be helpful if the child perceives the model as somewhat fearful but able to overcome his fears and cope adequately. If a model is perceived to be confident and masterful, he is less likely to influence the observer—"He may not be afraid, but I am."

Many practitioners have long used modeling strategies by letting the younger child watch "big sister" through the appointment if they perceive a positive relationship between a confident sibling and the fearful child. A simple variation of the same strategy involves scheduling an unrelated fearful child to watch another child patient during his appointment.

A more complex use of the strategy involving both the tell-show-do technique and modeling, but which can be successfully used by the practitioner, was described in 1971 by Papermaster, a pediatric dentist:

> A "leader" child, who has had dental work done previously, is seated in the dental chair. One of the new patients is asked to assist in making the dental examination. He is given the mouth mirror and (a blunted) explorer. ... Assist the child by holding his hand as he examines the teeth with the mouth mirror, checking the cavities and the fillings. He is then given the handpiece and is guided while one or two of the anterior teeth are polished with a rubber cup. He is given a pair of tweezers holding a piece of cotton and is asked to wipe off any particles on the teeth. The patient who has helped in the examination is then placed in the chair and another youngster is asked to help in the examination, and so on until all the children have been examined. Fillings are done for those who have previously visited the office, and the children are dismissed. After one or two Saturday morning appointments, these children can be taken care of at any time during the week in the same manner as any adult.

Parent in the Operatory?

This is a long-standing controversy, with strong feelings on both sides. In the past, most dentists treating children discouraged the parents' presence in the operatory (Roder *et al.*, 1961; Association of Pedodontic Diplomates, 1972 and 1981). However, it is no longer considered routine to exclude parents from the dental operatory (Musselman, 1991). Those who advocate keeping parents out argue that parents' presence disrupts procedures and provides an opportunity to communicate parental anxiety to the child. Those who advocate the parents' presence in the operatory suggest that the parent has a positive influence on increasing the security and coping of the young child in an unfamiliar environment. A number of non-dental studies support this position. The research conducted in the dental environment is limited and inconclusive. Two studies of prophylaxis, one assessing physiological responses (Lewis & Law, 1958), and the other assessing behavior (Allen & Evans, 1968), found no difference in children's responses when the parent either was or was not present. Similarly, Venham (1971) found no difference in the child's response to a series of two dental treatment visits, one with the mother present and one without. Frankl *et al.* (1962) found greater cooperative behavior during examination and subsequent treatment with the mother present. On the other hand, Croxton (1967) reported that of 28 children referred to his private practice because they had exhibited behavior problems at other dental offices, most had had treatment while a parent was present. As part of his treatment, he excluded parents and reported, by the final visit, a 93 percent success rate.

An interesting non-dental study by Shaw and Routh (1981) with a small number of children sheds additional light on this controversy. Eighteen-month and 5-year-old children received routine immunizations in a pediatrician's office with and without the mother present. Comparisons between conditions indicate that the behavior of children of both ages was more negative when the mother was present than when she was not. When the mother was present, children cried longer after injections and continued to "fuss" more while being dressed and taken from the examination room. The findings were interpreted to mean that, given a stressful experience, children may inhibit protest if the mother is absent.

It is clear that parents should not be routinely excluded from the operatory. In a number of situations parents can enhance management and reduce fears. Young children are susceptible to a number of fears, including fear of the unknown, separation from parents, and abandonment. Children commonly show such behavior up to about age 4. Children who cling to their parents and do not respond to an attractive play environment and overtures by the dentist and assistant to enter the operatory should not be forced to enter the operatory alone. On the other hand, depending on the goals of the visit, it may be useful to have the child inhibit his protestation.

It is useful to try to determine how the mother will behave in the operatory. In a number of studies in dental and medical settings, maternal anxiety consistently has been associated with fear-related child responses. Venham (1979) described four broad categories of mothers. One group sat passively and remained uninvolved. A second group attempted to obtain cooperative behavior from the child with no attempt to reduce anxiety and fear. These mothers used a variety of approaches, including comments, threats, and physical intervention. A third group focused on the child's feelings and attempts to reduce upset through verbal reassurance and physical contact. A fourth group tried to both reduce upset and gain cooperation. Clearly, parental effectiveness varies. Observing the parent and child and determining the parent's anxiety level are useful when you must decide whether or not the parent will be helpful or detrimental. For example, many dentists provide instruction to parents on their role in the operatory (Rayman, 1987).

Enhancing a Sense of Control

While control is clearly an important variable in managing fear within dental and other medical settings, it may be *especially* important for children. Feeling trapped and vulnerable are common child perceptions in the dental chair that contribute to fear. It is important to allow the child some control. While parents and dentists need to be in charge, it is probably best for children if you allow them to exercise some influence over events imposed upon them. Children allowed to *feel* in control show less fear. It is not difficult to structure simple choices for children. "Would you like to begin (cleaning) here or there?" "I have banana and strawberry (fluoride), which would you like?" When allowing the child to decide, you must always follow through. Therefore, do not ask whether or not the child wants to have dental treatment.

Signal mechanisms may be an additional possibility: "Just raise your hand like this [dentist raises the appropriate hand in the desired manner] if anything bothers you." Although prompt verbal recognition of the signal is important, the dentist need not stop immediately. Kruper (1970) showed that an experimental mechanical signaling device, which allowed the child to inform the dentist when he was feeling discomfort, resulted in more cooperative behavior than was elicited from children who did not have the device. It is interesting to note that the presence of such mechanical signaling devices may result in more cooperation but the child may not use them very often (Corah, 1973). Giving the child the *option* to stop is what is important. Mirrors, especially large hand mirrors, offer children additional control in being able to see what is going on. Like adults, many children relish the idea.

Control for children may be especially important when procedures are painful or otherwise aversive to the child. Milgrom, Vignehsa, and Weinstein (1992), in a study of Singapore adolescents, found that teens who reported painful treatment *and* perceived lack of control were 13.7 times more likely to report high dental fear. They were 15.9 times less likely to be willing to return to the dental environment than those who did not meet those conditions.

Techniques discussed in this section are useful, not only for children, but also for fearful adults. Slow and careful introduction of fearful adults to the dental environment, tell-show-do, modeling, allowing supportive friends and family into the operatory, establishing rapport and communication, and allowing some patient control are techniques that we recommend for *all* fearful patients.

Helping Children Cope

While the research literature on children's coping with fearful and painful situations is small, the same techniques useful to help adults cope may be slightly modified for use with children. For example, Heitkemper, Layne and Sullivan (1993) found a child's version of paced breathing to be especially effective in lowering anxiety and expected discomfort from dental treatment. We believe that *all anxious children should receive some instruction on how to cope.* Most children who are anxious can benefit from a few minutes of age-appropriate relaxation or breathing instruction. The following instructions present simple muscle relaxation and breathing exercises for preschool children that may be easily adapted for use with older children:

> I have a "Raggedy Ann" doll hanging on my wall. Sometimes when I want to get my body to feel more comfortable I put my body in the position of the doll. I make believe I'm the doll ... just hanging ... comfortable ... loose and limp. Let's think hard about one part of the body at a time ... Let's try your left arm. Imagine your arm just hanging... floppy ... like a Raggedy Ann doll's arm ... loose ... warm, limp ... So comfortable ...

The clinician models the relaxation exercise for the child and for the parent who may coach the child, and takes them through all four limbs and neck. Eyes may be open or closed.

> I have this nice balloon, I would like to blow up for you. [Begin blowing up balloon, but let it slip away as you are blowing it up. Do this twice or so.] Now stop laughing, you're not supposed to be having a good time here! What sound did the balloon make when it slipped away? ... It made a "sss" sound. Can you make this "sss" sound with me? ... Now take a big breath like this; hold it for a moment and then make the "sss" sound. Mom, I like to count with my fingers to help pace the breathing ... 1, 2, 3, 4, 5. Take another breath. I want you both to practice for a few minutes now. Any questions?

Very often we ask parents and children to practice these exercises at home. For older, school age children we use different images. For example:

> Do you have a bicycle? ... Tell me about it? ... Did you ever get a flat tire? ... What did it sound like? ... "sss?" ... Can you make this sound with me? ...

These techniques are distracting and somewhat hypnotic. At times a guided imagery or story-telling technique can be easily added to the exercise. The story may be completely improvised or may reflect an established theme, such as a child's television program, movie, or amusing or special activity. Encourage the child to contribute to the story. Use humor. For example, tell a familiar story, but do it the wrong way. Riding bicycles, magic carpet rides, birthday parties, cloud gazing, and racing cars or motorcycles are all possible. The Gardner and Olness text, *Hypnosis and Hypnotherapy with Children* (1981) provides instruction and many examples of useful techniques.

EFFECTIVE MANAGEMENT IN THE OPERATORY

The Guidance-Cooperation Model: A Useful Framework for Interaction with Children

An overall model of the practitioner—child interaction may be useful in conceptualizing your role and guiding your selection of child management strategies. The following model is derived from the work of two researchers whose contributions have broad application to all health care fields. In an article published in 1956, Szasz and Hollender identified three distinct models of doctor-patient relationships: the active-passive, guidance-cooperation, and mutual participation models.

We believe the dental practitioner-child relationship is best characterized as "guidance-cooperation." In this model the patient is not completely passive, as is the case in surgery where general anesthesia is required (the active-passive model). Neither is the child permitted to participate with the practitioner in making decisions about the dental procedure to be used (the mutual participation model). In a treatment situation characterized by guidance-cooperation, the child is expected to look up to and obey the practitioner. This model has its prototype in the relationship of parent and child and is especially relevant for pedodontics, where the practitioner is in a helping relationship with a young child. Research conducted in 1978 at the University of Washington School of Dentistry Pediatric Dentistry Clinic has indicated that the use of "directive guidance," a straightforward assertive statement of expectation with feedback concerning the child's behavior, led to cooperative child behavior. For example: "Open a little wider, please—good boy!" On the other hand, permissive behavior, such as saying, "Are you ready for me to begin now? Pretty please?" and coercive behavior, such as threats of scolding, resulted in substantial resistant and uncooperative child behavior (Wurster *et al.*, 1979).

A Study of Child Management

Subsequently, we undertook a major study of how children are managed in community dental offices. The major goal of the study was to identify effective and ineffective patterns of interaction between dentist and child and assistant and child. Twenty-five dentists volunteered. Fifty regular child patients of those dentists participated. Dentists identified 3- to 5-year-old children in their practices. These children were then screened by the dentist during their next appointment. Children who needed treatment requiring two or more sessions in which injections would be necessary were eligible for participation in the study.

Dentists agreed to avoid using nitrous oxide or any other pre-medication. Aside from this prohibition, they were asked to treat the child as they ordinarily would. All sessions were videotaped by an experienced technician. We analyzed 72 usable videotapes from 23 offices (Weinstein *et al.*, 1982).

A reliable but complex coding scheme was developed to help us analyze the data. Dimensions of child behavior included Movement and Physical Positioning, Verbal Behavior, and Comfort. Behaviors within these dimensions—for example, crying, discomfort, and inappropriate movement—were combined into fear and non-fear-related categories. Dentist and assistant dimensions included various forms of behavior coded as guidance-directs, explains, sets rules, coaxes, empathizes, i.e., questions about feelings, reassures, etc.; physical control and verbalization, i.e., silence, dental to child, distraction, etc.

To identify patterns of interaction between dentist and child and between assistant and child, we determined the probabilities that child fear-related behavior *followed* both dentist and assistant behavior. We did this for each procedure and for the appointment as a whole. Needless to say, the analysis was complex and required the use of a computer. On the other hand, the results were very easy to understand. We will discuss the most important results, one dimension at a time. First for the dentist, next for the assistant.

Effects of Dentist Behavior

When the dentist used directive guidance, fear-related behaviors were lowest after he used direction and reinforcement. Specific feedback (e.g., "You are doing a great job holding your head so still.") resulted in less fear-related behavior than general feedback (e.g., "You're being perfect."). Direction was more effective than rules, which are general directions given beforehand in anticipation of problem behavior; and rhetorical questions, e.g., "Could you open your mouth?" Young children respond to a rhetorical question as if it were a real question and not a social convention.

These findings clearly support learning theory, which states that the immediacy and strength of both discriminative stimuli (cues) and reinforcement (feedback) are important in understanding and controlling the behavior of the organism in the environment. Therefore, it was not surprising to find that rhetorical questions, such as "Would you like to get into the chair now?" (which are less immediate and strong), were much less effective in decreasing fear-related behaviors than specific direction.

Explanation was *not* the most effective technique with young children. Only during the low-stress chair placement phase did explanations precede a significant decrease in fear-related behaviors. Some support for this finding is found in the Howitt and Stricker (1965) work, which determined that "clarification" (explanation) was more effective with mildly anxious than highly anxious children. There is also evidence that information about anticipated events, such as surgery, may not decrease anxiety. Explanation is not a panacea. Three- to 5-year-old fearful children usually are not helped by rational discussion in fear providing situations. In fact, our clinical impression is that fearful children sometimes question and encourage explanation to avoid anticipated dental procedures.

Coercion (threats) and coaxing (pleas) are ineffectual management procedures. Dentists seem to use these procedures when they are frustrated by the child. Often the dentist's voice indicates his frustration, which may further exacerbate the situation. Emotional reactions are usually reciprocal: the child's fear-related behavior (stimulus) uses the dentist's frustration (response), which in turn causes further fear-related behavior in the child (stimulus). We hypothesize that by the time the dentist resorts to coercion and coaxing, he has already lost control of the situation.

In addition, a preschool child's ability to inhibit his own behaviors on demand is somewhat limited. Guidance to do something is usually more successful in getting the desired results than is a message to stop or slow down a behavior. Therefore, clinicians should focus on what they want the child to do. Inhibiting ongoing behavior is especially problematic with young children. It is better to prevent the problems before they emerge.

Questioning for feeling, e.g., "Tell me if anything is bothering you," which attempts to elicit and recognize the child's feelings, appears to be an effective dentist behavior. Reassurance, which may deny or ignore feelings, "Everything will be okay, don't worry," is followed by a greater probability of fear-related behavior. Reassurance, as Bernstein and associates (1974) have noted, does not really reassure. Analysis of dentists' empathy responses shows that reassurances were used most frequently during injection, rubber dam, and drilling phases, with very few occurrences recorded in earlier phases. Reassurances are used most frequently in stressful situations and have little effect in reducing fear.

These results support the position of Rogers (1961), who has long held that empathetic understanding—a combination of listening for another's feelings and expressing concern for those feelings—is a critical ingredient in helping relationships. Understanding makes the dentist aware of the patient's perception of dental procedures. In turn, the patient is more willing to trust the clinician, which influences how the patient structures the situation psychologically and how he subsequently responds.

Put-downs and ignoring or denying fear-related behaviors are ineffective and should be avoided. Interestingly, such behaviors resulted in a pattern similar to that found in extinction curves; when reinforcement is withheld, behavior does not dramatically decrease but decreases slowly. Such dentist behaviors may contribute to the etiology of phobias (see Chapter 2).

Other studies indicate that patting the child, a warm nonverbal gesture, is useful in reducing fear-related behavior in young children. And child management procedures such as directing, explaining, reinforcing, distracting, or reassuring are more effective when the dentist is in working contact with the child. Stopping dental procedures to manage child behavior is less effective. In such situations, halting treatment may inadvertently reinforce the child's fear-related behaviors. That is, the dentist rewards the child for fear-related behaviors by stopping the treatment.

Distracting young children does not appear to be an extremely useful approach. It is especially poor during the rubber dam application. After an injection, children are generally wary. The may perceive distraction at that time as a cue that another stressful procedure lies ahead.

In all, the evidence suggests that providing immediate direction and specific reinforcement are most consistently followed by a reduction in the child's fear-related behaviors. Patting and stroking also tend to be followed by a lessening of fear. Questioning for feeling is a useful technique; ignoring or denying a child's feelings is not. Coercion, coaxing, and put-downs tend to be followed by a substantial increase in fear-related responses by the child. Explanations, although frequently used, do not appear to significantly reduce fear-related responses. Moreover, stopping treatment *during treatment* to manage the child appears to result in more fear-related behaviors.

In addition, in a controlled study of nitrous oxide or placebo gas, Weinstein, Domoto, and Holleman (1986) found that the dentist's behavior was a major influence on the fear-related behaviors. Although a pharmacologic approach may be effective, the moment-by-moment patterns of interactions with children may determine the success of the appointment. Certain dentist behaviors, such as using suggestion, appear to be especially effective when nitrous oxide is being administered.

General Principles of Child Management

A number of general principles emerge from our work and that of our colleagues who study child management.

The Positive "What To Do"

Teach Simple Coping. Give anxious children a strategy they can use to keep themselves comfortable during dental treatment.

Use Specific Direction Giving. Use direct and specific requests for cooperation: "Please open your mouth, now"; "Turn this way; open a little wider"; "Put your hands back into your lap." Give the child the directions throughout the appointment and let him know what you expect him to do and not to do, i.e., "Keep your hands on your lap until I tell you it's O.K. to move again," or "Keep your head still, please, until I finish with this part."

Praise All Cooperative Behaviors. You cannot praise or "stroke" the child too frequently. When the child makes any attempt to respond to a directive, e.g., "open wide," praise him. Most important, do not forget to praise him when he is sitting still and cooperating. Much too often, we do not pay attention to the child until his behavior causes problems.

Use Specific Reinforcement. Express positive feelings to the patient for his cooperation, and explain *exactly* what she did that you found helpful. This technique is one of the single most effective procedures you can use to elicit cooperation. All of us, particularly children, like to know when we "do good."

"It really helps when you hold so still ... Good helping."

"You follow my directions very well, I appreciate that."

"Holding your head like that helps me get done much faster!"

"I like it when you hold your mouth open so wide. You make it easy for me."

General reinforcement expresses positive feelings to the patient for cooperation, but it does not specify a particular behavior. For example:

"You are a great patient."

"You're doing just fine."

"Good patient."

"That-a-girl."

Everyone likes to receive some general reinforcement occasionally. However, it is not nearly as effective as specific reinforcement in obtaining cooperation from a patient, because she can only guess what she was doing that pleases you.

Express Your Concern for the Child. Ask the child how he is feeling or if he is comfortable. Demonstrating your concern for the child is important to him. Verbal demonstration, e.g., "Are you okay?" "Is it too tight?" and eliciting signal mechanisms, e.g., "I want you to raise your hand if something is bothering you," are excellent management practices. A pat, a comforting gesture, is often appreciated.

Keep Your Cool. To show anger in response to a child's behavior will only make matters worse. If you can ignore irritating but non-interfering behavior such as crying or whining, do so. If you cannot, do not retaliate with coercion. We are not saying that you should not show your displeasure. A statement like, "I get mad (or unhappy, etc.) when you ...," when said in a calm voice, is more likely to succeed than coercion or permissiveness.

Use Voice Control. Use a sudden change in tone or volume to gain the attention of a child who is not cooperating. What you say is not critical; it is the change of voice that gains the child's attention. Return to the previous tone or volume as soon as the child begins to respond to your voice change. Again, do not show anger.

Allow the Child to Play a Role. Give the child a sense of control. Structure choices for her to make. For example, "Shall we count the top or bottom teeth first?" "Would you like me to help you into the chair or would you like to climb up yourself?" Most children want to be as adult as possible and enjoy the role of "helper." Helpers hold mirrors, swabs, etc., and receive praise for the good work they do. This is especially useful for preschoolers.

Structure Time. Specifying the amount of time that the child will spend in the chair may be useful, because it allows the fearful patient to pace himself. Knowledge that an invasive procedure will last only to a count of ten, or that only one minute is left before a procedure ends or a break occurs, can be very helpful. Sometimes we also show children an egg timer and negotiate in-chair time, after which they will be able to play with toys in the waiting room while you perform other duties.

Use Positive Suggestions. The role of suggestion describing and predicting future events in effective patient management is an important but almost totally unstudied topic. Neilburger (1978) presents a clinical investigation in children's dentistry. He compared the effect of suggestion, "When I brush your teeth it will tickle and make you laugh even more. You don't have to laugh too much, but many children do," to no suggestion, "Hello, Billy. How are you? Today we are going to clean your teeth with a magic toothbrush and toothpaste." Results indicated that suggestion decreased resistant behaviors. The most positive reaction was found among 6- to 8-year-old children.

The Negative: What to Avoid

Avoid Coercion, Belittlement, and Permissiveness. All are really very similar. They indicate to the child that you are ineffective in managing her behavior. They make things worse.

Avoid Elaborate Explanations. They are not important, especially after you have begun the treatment. Do not try to talk a child into cooperation. Explain while you work, do not stop to explain, and do not get caught up in responding to a barrage of questions. Tell the child you will respond to questions after the treatment and live up to your promise.

Do Not Rely Heavily on Rule-Setting or Distraction. Both have limited effectiveness. Distraction, as a dentist-initiated strategy to control child anxiety, probably should not be used after the initial injection. Children learn quickly. On the other hand, distraction can be used as a child coping strategy.

Avoid Premature Reassurance. "It's going to be O.K.," "It won't bother you for very long," "There, that wasn't so bad," "Almost done, just a little longer," are, at best, overused. They tend to be ineffective. When a child protests, you can express empathy and understanding by saying something like, "I know you don't really want to be here," (or "like this part"), or "I wish you didn't have to do this too, *but* when you are at the dentist's, there are lots of funny things you have to do that you don't do anywhere else. So let's get on with it and finish. Then we can go and do something else." Then in a firm but calm voice, continue with a specific direction or command.

Avoid Relying on a Drug as the Primary Means to Manage the Child. We will discuss pharmacological agents later in this chapter. While drugs can be useful adjuncts for managing anxiety, they are rarely a substitute for effective behavioral management of the child in a community practice. The primary approach must be behavioral.

Effects of Assistant Behavior

Results of our work have implications for the assistant's role in child management (Weinstein *et al.*, 1983). Gently holding the child *before* disruptive movement and restraining appears to be a well accepted and effective assistant behavior in managing difficult children.

Others, e.g., reinforcement of positive behavior and questioning for feeling, appear to be used by assistants with some effectiveness. Surprisingly, assistant pats were found to be ineffective. This may be because pats are given only when the child is already showing fear and are not used in prevention.

Other factors that influence assistant behavior have also been explored. Though the correlations were only moderate between assistant and dentist behaviors, additional analyses of behavior patterns reveal that assistants look to dentists to model behavior. Unfortunately, dentist control of the situation, though essential, has caused auxiliaries to play less than optimal roles. We agree with Starkey (1975) that "the dental auxiliary must understand, accept and share the philosophy of the dentist; otherwise, she will be unable to support him..." There is much to be gained by enhancing the assistant's support role in this area, and there may be a need for formal instruction to develop the role in dental assisting programs. At the very least, a structured inservice training or orientation program is indicated.

Treating the Older Child and Teenager

Although most of what we have written focuses on the fear-related behaviors of the young child, older children and adolescents can also be fearful. Fear in the older child often seems to center on the injection. Many of these children are old enough to travel to their appointments independently. No-shows are a frequent problem. With these children, age 10+, we usually expect too much. The natural tendency is to treat the physically mature child as if he were socially and mentally mature. In reality, the huge 12-year-old may have the emotional control of a 6-year-old, whereas a childlike wisp of a prepubescent teenager may show the mental maturity of a young adult.

Flexibility and frustration tolerance are therefore important for the clinician. We try, by trial and error, to communicate effectively. We are careful not to enter into the dynamics of any ongoing developmental difficulties. This means that we do *not* take on the parental role. We try to establish and maintain a personal relationship with these children that is independent of the parent. When they do not meet our expectations, e.g., they fail to show up for appointments or otherwise do not agree to work on their fears with us, we do not punish them, verbally or otherwise. Anger is counter-productive. These children are frequently yelled at by parents, teachers, and other adults. Their day is filled with coercion; their response is resistance, passive or otherwise.

We communicate with these children in an adult-to-adult manner. Rapport may be difficult to establish, because the child may not respond to our conversation. We encourage *all* verbalizations with children who are silent by giving many positive verbal strokes for the most meager utterances. We try to show the child that we like him.

At an early point, we discuss with the child whether or not he wants to overcome his fears and to receive treatment. We present a treatment plan not only to the parent, or parent and child together, but also to the child alone. We make it clear that he has ultimate decisional and behavioral control over all dental events and that we are working for *him*, even though his parents are paying the freight. It is his body. We will go at his speed.

We also tell him that we recognize that coming here and facing his fears is work. He deserves to feel proud and be rewarded. We choose a regular time for appointments. We recommend that parent, child, and dentist enter into a contractual agreement about attending sessions and completing homework assignments, if needed. For example, after two missed appointments with a 16 year old, we negotiated an agreement that his mother would give us $5.00 per completed appointment, to be exchanged for a much desired fishing reel for the child after treatment was completed. Moreover, charges for missed appointments were to be paid for by the parent *and* the fund established to buy the reel.

If a parent expresses concern over "bribing" the child, it will be necessary to clarify the difference between bribery and reinforcement. A "bribe" is defined as something offered to induce dishonest acts. Reinforcement is used to teach appropriate behaviors; it is used temporarily because the behavior does not, at the time, have intrinsic reward.

Aversive Management Techniques and Alternatives

There is a class of child management procedures that cause children, and us, discomfort. These techniques are primarily oriented toward forcing compliance, not managing fear. The techniques in this category include strapping the child down or wrapping him in a sheet and placing a hand over his mouth (HOM), and perhaps his nose as well.

In a 1980 survey of attitudes and practices of members of the American Academy of Pedodontics, almost 98 percent of all members, including Diplomates, used "hand over mouth" in selected cases. The purposes included gaining cooperation and attention and "dampening vocal noise." Other restraints were used in selected cases by 86 percent of the members. A more recent survey indicated that the use of airway blocking techniques, especially techniques that are extremely aversive, i.e., covering both airways, are being taught less often and that there is a trend for new directors of graduate programs to rely less on airway restriction (Acs *et al.*, 1990). It appears that these techniques are out-of-date. Casamassino noted in his 1993 editorial that "Our society is moving to eliminate HOM from the behavioral armamentarium ..."

We think it is unfortunate that so many clinicians use some form of aversive management when a positive management approach fails. Such action indicates low tolerance for children's demonstration of upset and fear and a procedure-oriented practice philosophy. We see a number of adults in the Dental Fears Research Clinic who were abused by these techniques when they were children. When reaching adulthood, these people avoid dental care almost completely. Such procedures perpetuate negative stereotypes of dentists. *Hand over mouth and other restraints should not be used in dental practice, except during an emergency.* Using aversive techniques so that a prophylaxis or a restoration can be accomplished is not warranted. Few parents, if given a choice, would consent to such procedures. It is our bet that dentists who rely heavily on such procedures do so without parents in the operatory. Recently, after considerable debate, professional guidelines require written informed consent before such procedures may be used.

Hand-over-mouth technique has been used for over 50 years. Most advocates specify that the technique is a last resort, to be used to establish communication after all other approaches have failed and the child's behavior remains uncontrolled. Even advocates warn that the technique, which involves removing the clinician's hand from the child's mouth only when the child cooperates, is contra-indicated for children under age three, for those who are mentally impaired, and for children who have been sedated. Moreover, there are numerous other caveats, the most important being that the clinician not behave emotionally; he must control his own response. This is most difficult; techniques of last resort are not readily used without emotion, especially when the dentist is frustrated and angry. The scenario of a screaming, flailing child is emotionally charged. Children can sense the clinician's anger and inadequacy and they do not respond positively in such situations.

Alternatives

Alternative strategies do exist. We have found that aversive tech-niques are often used prematurely. Children do not show tantrum behavior or try to flee in the chair without warning. They show numerous signs of fear and upset, which the dentist usually ignores or responds to by superficial reassurance. Often, the clinician does not take enough time to establish rapport and to reinforce positive behaviors. Moreover, he usually wants to complete procedures with-in a given period of time. Stopping or not completing a procedure is viewed as a defeat and is intolerable to some dentists. *Ending a procedure when a child is getting tired or upset is a good idea.* In doing so we close the appointment on a positive note and praise the child for whatever cooperation he has shown. In some circumstances, we have praised the child for just sitting in the chair. Allen *et al.* (1991) reported a successful variation of this technique in which children aged 3 to 7 were allowed to temporarily escape after brief periods of cooperative behavior.

When the child begins to panic, scream or flail, there is little that we can do to manage his fear effectively. It is too late. The child should be told that he has done well and that we are done for the day. The following appointment should build coping skills, include a rehearsal, and have modest goals—the child should have consider-able positive verbal reinforcement for any bit of cooperation, and play interspersed with treatment.

At times desensitization may be necessary. One caveat—children often do very well with this approach but are not capable of indicat-ing to the clinician that they are ready for an aversive procedure such as an injection. Sometimes we have the child raise her hand only if she does *not* want to go ahead. Other times we have the child delegate the responsibility of deciding when to go ahead to a trusted adult. Using pharmacological agents is a distinct possibility and will be discussed in this chapter. The modeling of other siblings and friends is another alternative. Clearly, the parent must understand what is going on and be part of the decision-making. Treatment of this sort is more costly than hand-over-mouth, but worth the expense in the long run.

PHARMACOLOGICAL MANAGEMENT TECHNIQUES

There is no drug available to general practitioners that will obtund a child to the extent that it can substitute fully for the behavioral techniques discussed earlier. The child's anxious or uncooperative behavior may, in fact, be worse under inadequate sedation than if the child had full control. Thus, we must temper recommendations regarding the use of pharmacological agents.

At the outset we also need to recognize the importance of pain control during treatment of children. In general there has been under-recognition of this need and it is often mixed up with child behavior management. In a survey of Seattle dentists we found that one in three did not routinely use local anesthetics when doing restorations or extractions. A similar proportion did not routinely provide post-operative pain medications after tooth extractions. These practices were shown to be negatively related to the dentist's comfort treating children and his need to control the child's behavior. A surprising proportion of dentists routinely deny child pain responses (Milgrom *et al.*, 1994). Yet children are generally good reporters of pain (McGrath, 1990).

Good technique is essential for painless and effective analgesia with children. Topical analgesia should always be used. Benzocaine or similar drugs, usually in ointment form, are effective. They have rapid onset (1-2 minutes) and fairly long duration. They also have very limited toxicity or allergy potential. These viscous materials can be applied on a cotton roll left in place or on a cotton swab. One has to be cautious to avoid getting the topical everywhere and alarming the child. Similarly, liquids and sprays are hard to control.

The dentist should taste the preparation himself to know how to avoid unpleasant materials. Recently, one author suggested that EMLA cream (a mixture of local anesthetics), used quite effectively in children's hospitals for skin anesthesia, might also be useful in the mouth. However effective, the onset is fairly slow (Svensson & Petersen, 1992).

There is much lore about painless injections. The key factors appear to be topical analgesia, blanching pressure on the tissue, and slow injection. A rate of 1 ml per minute is appropriate. Most dentists need to time themselves to learn to proceed that slowly. It is beyond the scope of this text to address specific pharmacological issues regarding doses. We refer readers to current texts in pediatric dentistry and pharmacology (e.g., Neidle & Yagiela, 1989). Nevertheless, for a child exceeding 100 pounds (45 kg) the adult maximums apply. For smaller children, the maximum safe doses are, for standard anesthetics with a vasoconstrictor, 6-7 mg/kg. The maximum safe dose for Lidocaine without a vasoconstrictor is about one-half of that with a vasoconstrictor (Petersen & Milgrom, 1989). Anesthetic doses may need to be reduced when sedative, narcotic or antiemetic drugs are also used (Goodson & Moore, 1983) or where there are other health problems.

For post-operative pain control, liquid acetaminophen (paracetemol) is the drug of choice for small children. Doses should range from 60-120 mg/kg in children one to six and 150-300 mg/kg for older children up to age 12. Salicylates are generally avoided in children (Neidle & Yagiela, 1989).

Sedative Hypnotics

A number of drugs have been marketed for pediatric sedation and used in pediatric dentistry. Many have been withdrawn because of safety concerns, and surprisingly, few of the recommendations in the literature are really based on placebo-controlled clinical trials. This is because drug companies have been reluctant to incur the liability risk associated with trials specifically with children and because such trials are difficult to conduct. A team of investigators at the Dental Fears Research Clinic has been active in trying to remedy this situation.

One agent well tested at the University of Washington in controlled, double blind trials sponsored by the National Institute of Dental Research, is nitrous oxide (Weinstein *et al.*, 1986). If a child appears anxious or did not do well in previous appointments, it is appropriate to assess the potential of nitrous oxide in tandem with good behavioral technique to ameliorate his anxiety. This assessment should be independent of any dental treatment. At an appointment where no dental work is planned, see if the child will accept the nose piece, usually placed without the restraining hoses. If the child will accept the nose piece, then a short session where he is exposed to 30 percent nitrous oxide and practices deep breathing is appropriate. Only after it is clear that the child accepts the drug should it be used in conjunction with dental treatment.

The drug most cited in the pediatric dentistry literature is chloral hydrate (Noctec®, Duncan *et al.*, 1983). This drug will often be ineffective if not combined with behavioral techniques. It should be used only after you carefully assess the effectiveness of other approaches. The agent is a non-barbiturate sedative hypnotic available as a 500 mg/5 ml syrup. Typically it is used at a dose of 50 mg/kg up to 1 g. It maybe used in conjunction with nitrous oxide, hydroxyzine (1 mg/kg), or promethazine (1 mg/kg). It has a half-life of four to 12 hours. The literature, however, is somewhat misleading. Claims have been made that chloral hydrate is safer than short-acting barbiturates, no longer used in dentistry. In fact, there is no difference in the therapeutic index. Severe laryngospasm with cardiorespiratory arrest have been reported. Dose dependent depression is found. Moreover, a severely anxious and upset child will require very large doses to obtund the uncooperative behavior, rendering the use of the drug unsafe outside of hospital settings. Be especially cautious when combining chloral hydrate and other drugs, particularly local anesthetic, because peri-operative mortality has been reported in dental cases (Goodson & Moore, 1983). Nonetheless, chloral hydrate is a pharmacological agent worth having available.

Newer approaches to using pharmacological agents involve the benzodiazepines. As with other drugs, there have been few clinical trials and no placebo-controlled trials that meet international standards. With the exception of diazepam, none of these drugs are specifically licensed for use with children in the U.S. Diazepam may be used as a premedicant at a dose of 0.2 to 0.5 mg/kg. It has a one-hour onset. Triazolam (Halcion®, 0.015 to 0.025 mg/kg) has been demonstrated as a safe agent both in outpatient and hospital settings (Quarnstrom *et al.*, 1992). It can be suspended effectively in Kool-Aid or the small tablet can be crushed and mixed in food. Its onset is about 30 minutes. In order to be consistently effective, drug use needs to be combined with good behavioral technique. Drugs alone have mixed efficacy.

We badly need good research on sedative agents for children and their effects. The Dental Fears Research Clinic, in conjunction with the Department of Anesthesiology of the University of Washington School of Medicine, has recently received FDA approval to begin studies in this area. With all sedative agents, safety is paramount. Children should never be left unattended and careful airway management is essential. All staff members should have appropriate CPR training and emergency procedures should be well established. Essential emergency equipment should be available and in proper working order. Where required by state laws, everyone should be licensed to use these agents.

CONCLUSION

In all, we have discussed a wide variety of child management procedures. For the child, the dental office may be an unfamiliar or threatening environment. Altering the child's perceptions, through careful introduction to dentistry and attention to communication itself, will yield cooperative children with minimal fear. In the long run, the preventive approach is most efficient.

Creating a safe atmosphere for children is the goal of our efforts. Preventive efforts worth taking include establishing rapport and communication and giving the child a sense of control. Careful introduction of the child to the dental environment is helpful. Positive management of the child involves minimizing coercion, coaxing, premature verbal reassurance, and other such behaviors, while teaching the child how to cope and maximizing direction, feedback, and emphatic behaviors such as questioning for feelings. While they are under-utilized in behavior management, there are effective behavior guidelines for assistants. When a positive approach fails, hand-over-mouth and other aversive procedures are not generally warranted. Alternative procedures, including a range of pharmacologic adjuncts, can often be substituted effectively.

QUESTIONS AND EXERCISES

1. Consider the preappointment letter. Can you think of any changes you would make in this to fit your own style or office practice? If so, draft such a letter.

2. Reflecting on the origins of dental fear, consider how each child management strategy described here could help to prevent the development of fear.

3. Develop a list of phrases that you can use in various situations, e.g., putting on the rubber dam, which (a) convey interest and empathy for children, (b) can reinforce specific behaviors, and (c) give specific and clear directions that will be unambiguous for children of different ages.

4. How can you give a child patient a sense of control? Give specific examples.

5. Practice teaching a child a coping skill. Try a five year old and an older child.

6. Describe the guidelines for your child practice on the use of nitrous oxide and other pharmacological agents. How would you introduce nitrous oxide to a six year old who needs restorative care?

7. Under what circumstances would you ask a mother to remain in the waiting room?

Bibliography

Acs, G., Burke, M.J., and Musson, C.M. An updated survey on the utilization of hand over mouth (HOM) and restraint in postdoctoral pediatric dental education. *Pediatric Dentistry* 1990; *12*:298–302.

Addelston, K.K. Child patient training. *Fortnightly Review of the Chicago Dental Society* 1959; *38*:7–11.

Agras, S., Sylvester, D., and Oliveau, D. The epidemiology of common fears and phobia. *Comprehensive Psychiatry* 1979; *10*:151–56.

Allen, B.P. and Evans, R.I. Video tape recording in social psychological research: an illustrative study of pedodontia. *Psychological Reports* 1968; *23*:1115–19.

Allen, K.D., Loiben, T., Allen, S.J., and Stanley, R.T. Dentist-implemented contingent escape for management of disruptive child behavior. *Journal of Applied Behavior Analyses* 1992; *25*:629–36.

Allen, W.A. In P. Sykes (Ed.), *Dental sedation and anesthesia.* London, SAAD, 1979.

Alvesalo, I., Murtomaa, H., Milgrom, P., Honkanen, A., Karjalainen, M., and Tay, K-M. The Dental Fear Survey Schedule: a study with Finnish children. *International Journal of Pediatric Dentistry* 1993; *3*:15–20.

American Dental Association. *Accepted Dental Therapeutics* 41st ed., Chicago: American Dental Association, September (1982).

American Psychiatric Association. *Diagnostic and statistical manual of mental disorders* (Third Edition—Revised) Washington, D.C.: American Psychiatric Association Press, 1987.

Association of Pedodontic Diplomates. Technique for behavior management A survey. *Journal of Dentistry for Children* 1972; *39*:368–72.

Association of Pedodontic Diplomates. Survey of attitudes and practices in behavior management. *Pediatric Dentistry* 1981; *3*:246–50.

Auerbach, S.M., Kendall, P.C., Cuttler, H.F., and Levitt, N.R. Anxiety, locus of control, type of preparatory information and adjustment to dental treatment. *Journal of Consulting and Clinical Psychology* 1976; *44*:809–18.

Averill, J.R. Personal control over aversive stimuli and its relationship to stress. *Psychological Bulletin* 1973; *80*:286–303.

Baab, D. and Weinstein, P. Oral hygiene instruction using a self-inspection index. *Community Dentistry and Oral Epidemiology* 1983; *11*:174–79.

Babajews, A.V. and Ivanyi, L. The relationship between in vivo and in vitro reactivity of patients with a history of allergy to local anesthetics. *British Dental Journal* 1982; *152*(11):385–87.

Bailey, P.M., Talbot, A., and Taylor, P.P. A comparison of maternal anxiety levels with anxiety levels manifested in the child dental patient. *Journal of Dentistry for Children* 1978; *45*:62–67.

Bandura, A. Self-efficacy: toward a unified theory of behavioral change. *Psychological Review* 1977; *84*:191–215.

Barash, D.P. Human ethology: displacement activities in a dental office. *Psychological Reports* 1974; *34*:947–49.

Barber, T.X. Physiological effects of "hypnotic suggestions." A critical review of recent research (1960–64). *Psychological Bulletin* 1965; *63*:201–22.

Barenie, J.T. Inhalation conscious sedation: Nitrous oxide analgesia. In L.W. Ripa and J.T. Barenie (Eds.), *Management of dental behavior in children*. Littleton, Massachusetts: PSG Publishing Co., 1979.

Baron, R.S., Logan, H., and Hoppe. Emotional and sensory focus as mediators of dental pain among patients differing in desired and felt dental control. *Health Psychology* 1993; *12*(5):381–89.

Beck, A.T. *Cognitive therapy and emotional disorders.* New York: New American Library, 1979.

Bedi, R., Sutcliffe, P., Donnan, P.T., and McConnachie, J. The prevalence of dental anxiety in a group of 13- and 14-year old Scottish children. *International Journal of Paediatric Dentistry* 1992; *2*:17–24.

Bergendal, B. The relative importance of tooth loss and denture wearing in Swedish adults. *Community Dental Health* 1989; *6*:103–11.

Berger, D.E. Assessment of the analgesic effects of nitrous oxide on the primary dentition. *Journal of Dentistry for Children* 1972; *39*:265–68.

Berggren, U. Dental fear and avoidance. A study of etiology, consequences and treatment. Published doctoral thesis, Faculty of Odontology, University of Göteborg, Sweden, 1984.

Berggren, U. and Lindhe, A. Dental fear and avoidance: A compari son of two modes of treatment. *Journal of Dental Research* 1984; 63:1223–27.

Bernstein, D.A., Kleinknecht, R.A., and Alexander, L.D. Antecedents of dental fear. *Journal of Public Health Dentistry* 1979; 39:113–24.

Bernstein, D.A. and Kleinknecht, R.A. Multiple approaches to the reduction of dental fear. *Journal of Behavior Therapy and Experimental Psychology* 1982; 13:187–92.

Bernstein, L., Bernstein, R.S., and Dana, R.H. *Interviewing: A guide for health professionals.* New York: Appleton-Century-Crofts, 1974.

Berthold, C.W., Schneider, A., and Dionne, R.A. Using triazolam to reduce dental anxiety. *Journal of the American Dental Association* 1993; 124:58–64.

Bolles, R.C. and Fanselow, M.S. A perceptual-defensive-recuperative model of fear and pain. *The Behavioral and Brain Sciences* 1980; 3:291–323.

Borland, L.R. Odontophobia—inordinate fear of dental treatment. *Dental Clinics of North America* 1962; 6:683–695.

Brandon, R.K. and Kleinknecht, R.A. Fear assessment in a dental analogue setting. *Journal of Behavioral Assessment* 1982; 4:317–25.

Brauner, A. Reduktion von Angsten im Verlauf einer zahnarzlichen Behandllung. *Deutsche Zahnarztl Zeitschrift* 1989; 44:353–55.

Butler, J.H., Abbott, D.M., and Bush, F.M. Biofeedback as a method of controlling bruxism. *Journal of Dental Research* 1976; 55:B310.

Cannistraci, A. A method to control bruxism: biofeedback-assisted relaxation therapy. *Journal of the American Society for Preventive Dentistry* 1976; 6:12–15.

Cannon, W.B. *Bodily changes in pain, hunger, fear and rage* (2nd ed.). New York: Appleton-Century-Crofts, 1929.

Carlsson, S.G., Gale, E.N., and Ohman, A. Treatment of temporomandibular joint syndrome with biofeedback training. *Journal of the American Dental Association* 1975; 91:602–5.

Casamassimo, P.S. Maybe the last editorial on hand-over-mouth technique. *Pediatric Dentistry* 1993; 15:233.

Cesar, J., de Moraes, A.B.A., Milgrom, P., and Kleinknecht, R.A. Cross validation of a Brazilian version of the Dental Fear Survey. *Community Dentistry and Oral Epidemiology* 1993; 21:148–50.

Chaves, J.F. and Brown, J.M. Self-generated strategies for the control of pain and stress. Paper presented at the annual meeting of the

American Psychological Association, August 1978, Toronto, Canada.

Chellappah, N.K., Vignehsa, H., Milgrom, P., and Lo, G. Prevalence of dental anxiety and fear in children in Singapore. *Community Dentistry and Oral Epidemiology* 1990; *18*:269–71.

Clark D.M. A cognitive model of panic attacks. In S. Rachman and J. Maser (Eds.), *Panic: psychological perspectives*. Hilldale, New Jersey: Erlbaum, 1988.

Clum, G.A., Scott, L., and Burnside, J. Information and locus of control as factors in the outcome of surgery. *Psychological Reports* 1979; *45*:867–73.

Clum, G.A., Luscomb, R.L., and Scott, L. Relaxation training and cognitive redirection strategies in the treatment of acute pain. *Pain* 1982; *12*:175–83.

Connolly, J., Hallam, R.S., and Marks, I.M. Selective association of fainting with blood-injury-illness fear. *Behavior Therapy* 1976; *7*:8–13.

Corah, N.L. Assessment of a dental anxiety scale. *Journal of Dental Research* 1969; *43*:496.

Corah, N.L. Effect of perceived control on stress reduction in pedodontic patients. *Journal for Dental Research* 1973; *52*:1261–64.

Corah, N.L., Gale, E.N., and Illig, S.J. Psychological stress reduction during dental procedures. *Journal of Dental Research* 1979a ; *53*:1347–51.

Corah, N.L., Gale, E.N., and Illig, S.J.The use of relaxation and distraction to reduce psychological stress during dental procedures. *Journal of the American Dental Association* 1979b; *98*:388–94.

Corah, N.L. Relaxation and musical programming as a means of reducing psychological stress during dental procedures. *Journal of the American Dental Association* 1981; *103*:232–34.

Croxton, W.L. Child behavior and the dental experience. *Journal of Dentistry for Children* 1967; *34*:212–18.

Cumming, B.R. and Löe, H. Consistency of plaque distribution in individuals without special home care instruction. *Journal for Periodontal Research* 1973; *8*:94–100.

Davey, G.C.L. Dental phobias and anesthetics: Evidence for conditioning processes in the acquisition and modulation of learned fear. *Behaviour Research and Therapy* 1989; *27*:51–58.

Davison, G.C. and Neale, J.M. *Abnormal psychology*. New York: John Wiley and Sons, 1982.

De Jongh, A., Muris, P., ter Horst, G., Van Zuuren, F.J., and De Wit, C..A. Cognitive correlates of dental anxiety. *Journal of Dental Research* 1994; 73(2):561–66.

De Jongh, A., Stouthard, M.E. Anxiety about dental hygienist. *Community Dentistry and Oral Epidemiology* 1993; 21:91–95.

De Jongh, A., Stouthard, M.E.A., and Hoogstraten, J. Sex differences in dental anxiety. *Nederlands Tijdscrift voor Tandheelkunde* 1991; 98(4):156–57.

Devine, V., Adelson, R., Goldstein, J., Valins, S., and Davison, G.C. Controlled test of the analgesic and relaxant properties of nitrous oxide. *Journal for Dental Research* 1979; 53:486–90.

Dionne, R.A., Wirdzek, P.R., Fox, P.C., and Dubner, R. Suppression of postoperative pain by the combination and nonsteroidal anti-inflammatory drug, florbiprofen and a long acting local anesthetic, etidocaine. *Journal of the American Dental Association* 1984; 108:598–601.

Dionne, R.A. New approaches to preventing and treating postoperative pain. *Journal of the American Dental Association* 1992; 123:26–34.

Domoto, P.K., Weinstein, P., Melnick, S., Ohmura, M., Uchida, H., Ohmachi, K., Hori, M., Okazaki, Y., Shimamoto, T., Matsumura, S., and Shimono, T. Results of a dental fear survey in Japan: Implications for dental public health in Asia. *Community Dentistry and Oral Epidemiology* 1988; 16:199–201.

Duke, M.P. and Cohen, B. Locus of control as an indication of patient cooperation. *Journal of the American College of Dentistry* 1974; 41:174–78.

Duncan, W.K., Pruhs, R.J., Ashrafi, M.H., and Post, A.C. Choral hydrate and other drugs used in sedating young children: A survey of the American Academy of Pedodontics Diplomates. *Pediatric Dentistry* 1983; 5:252–56.

Dworkin, S.F., Chen, A.C., LeResche, L., Clark, D.W. Cognitive reversal of expected nitrous oxide analgesia for acute pain. *Anesthesia – analgesia* Dec. 1983; 62(12):1073–7.

Egbert, L.D., Battit, G.E., Welch, C.E., and Bartlett, M.K. Reduction of post-operative pain by encouragement and instruction of patients.

New England Journal of Medicine 1964; 270:825–27.

Egelberg, J. *Periodontics the scientific way: Synopses of human clinical studies.* Copenhagen: Munksgaard, 1992.

Eli, I. Dental anxiety: a cause for possible misdiagnosis of tooth vitality. *International Endodontic Journal* 1993; 26:251–53.

Elliott, R. Tonic heart rate: experiments in the effects of collative variables lead to a hypothesis about its motivational significance. *Journal of Personality and Social Psychology* 1969; 12:211–28.

Ellis, A. *A new guide to rational living.* North Hollywood, CA: Wilshire Books, 1975.

Emmertsen, E. The treatment of children under general analgesia. *Journal of Dentistry for Children* 1965; 32:123–24.

Enneking, D., Milgrom, P., Weinstein, P., and Getz, T. Treatment outcomes for specific subtypes of dental fear: preliminary clinical findings. *Special Care in Dentistry* 1992; 12:214–18.

Evans, R.I. Motivating changes in oral hygiene behavior: some social psychological perspectives. *Journal of Preventive Dentistry* 1978; 5:14–19.

Fink, M., Taylor, M.A., and Volavka, J. Anxiety precipitated by lactate. *New England Journal of Medicine* 1969; 281:1429.

Fiset, L., Milgrom, P., Weinstein, P., Getz, T., and Glassman, P. Psychophysiological responses to dental injections. *Journal of the American Dental Association* 1985; 111:578–83.

Fiset, L., Ramsay, D., Milgrom, P., and Weinstein, P. Effects of lidocaine with epinephrine on fear-related arousal among simple dental phobics undergoing tooth extraction. *Anesthesia Progress* 1986; 33(5):225–29.

Fiset, L., Getz, T., Milgrom, P., and Weinstein, P. Local anesthesia failure: Diagnosis and management strategies. *General Dentistry* 1989; Sept-Oct 37(5):414–17.

Fiset, L., Milgrom, P., Weinstein, P., and Melnick, S. Common fears and their relationship to dental fear and utilization of the dentist. *Anesthesia Progress* 1989; 36:258–64.

Fiset, L., Milgrom, P., Weinstein, P., and Yagiela, J.A. Exaggerated psychophysiological response to local anesthetics: report of two cases. *Journal of the American Analgesia Society* 1990; 24(1):11–13.

Fisher, G.C. Management of fear in the child patient. *Journal of the American Dental Association* 1958; 57:792–95.

Flor, H. and Birbaumer, N. Comparison of Electromyographic biofeedback, Cognitive-behavioral therapy and conservative medical interventions in the treatment of chronic musculoskeletal pain. *Journal of Consulting and Clinical Psychology* 1993; 61(4):653–58.

Folkman, S. and Lazarus, R.S. Coping in an adequately functioning middle aged population. *Journal of Health and Social Behavior* 1980; 21:219–39.

Fordyce, W.E. Behavioral Methods for Chronic Pain and Illness. St. Louis: C.V. Mosby, 1976.

Forehand, R.L. and McMahon, R.J. *Helping the noncompliant child.* New York: The Guilford Press, 1981.

Forgione, A.G. and Clark, R.E. Comments on an empirical study of the cause of dental fears. *Journal of Dental Research* 1974; 53:496.

Fox, E., O'Boyle, C., Barry, H., and McCreary, C. Repressive coping style and anxiety in stressful dental surgery. *British Journal of Medical Psychology* 1989; 62:371–80.

Frankl, S.N., Fogels, H.R., and Shiere, F.R. Should the parent remain with the child in the dental operatory? *Journal of Dentistry for Children* 1962; 29:150–63.

Frazer, M. and Hampson, S. Some personality factors related to dental anxiety and fear of pain. *British Dental Journal* 1988; 165;436–39.

Freidson, E. and Feldman, J.J. The public looks at dental care. *Journal of the American Dental Association* 1958; 57:325–35.

Friedman, N., Cecchini, J.J., Wexler, M., and Pitts, W.C. A dentist oriented fear reduction technique: the iatrosedative process. *Compendium* 1989; 10:113–14, 116–18.

Gale, E.N. and Ayer, W.A. Treatment of dental phobias. *Journal of the American Dental Association* 1969; 78:1304–07.

Gale, E. Fears of the dental situation. *Journal of Dental Research* 1972; 51:964–66.

Gardner, G.G. and Olness, K. *Hypnosis and hypnotherapy with children.* Philadelphia: Grune & Stratton, 1981.

Gardner, W.J. and Licklider, J.C.R. Auditory analgesia in dental operations. *Journal of the American Dental Association* 1959; 59:1144–49.

Gardner, W.J., Licklider, J.C.R., and Weisz, A.Z. Suppression of pain by sound. *Science* 1960; *132*:32–33.

Garzone, P.D. Kroboth, P.D. Pharmacokinetics of the newer benzo-diazepines. *Clinical Pharmacokinetics* 1989; *16*:337–64.

Gatchel, R.J. The prevalence of dental fear and avoidance: Expanded adult and recent adolescent surveys. *Journal of the American Dental Association* 1989; *118*:591–93.

Geer, J.H., Davison, G.C., and Gatchel, R.I. Reduction of stress in humans through nonveridical perceived control of aversive stimulation. *Journal of Personality and Social Psychology* 1970; *16*:731–38.

George, J.M., Scott, D.S., Turner, S.P., and Gregg, J.M. The effects of psychological factors and physical trauma on recovery from oral surgery. *Journal of Behavioral Medicine* 1980; *3*:291–300.

Glaros, A. and Gadbury–Amyot, C. How personal protective equipment affects perceptions of dentists *Journal of the American Dental Association* 1993; *124*(10):82–88.

Glennon, B. and Weisz, J.R. An observational approach to the assessment of anxiety in young children. *Journal of Consulting and Clinical Psychology* 1978; *46*:1246–57.

Gold, S.L. Establishing motivating relations in preventive dentistry. *Journal of the American Society of Preventive Dentistry* 1974; *4*:17–25.

Goodson, J..M. and Moore, P.A. Life threatening reactions after pediatric sedation: An assessment of narcotic, local anesthetic and antiemetic drug interaction. *Journal of the American Dental Association* 1983; *107*:239–45.

Hain, J.D., Butcher, H.G., and Stevenson, I. Systematic desensitization therapy: an analysis of results in twenty–seven patients. *British Journal of Psychiatry* 1966; *112*:297–307.

Hakeberg, M., Berggren, U., Carlsson, S.G. Prevalence of dental anxiety in an adult population in a major urban area in Sweden. *Community Dentistry and Oral Epidemiology* 1992; *20*:97–101.

Hall, N. and Edmonson, H.D. The aetiology and psychology of dental fear. *British Dental Journal* 1983; *154*:247–52.

Hawley, B.P., McCorkle, A.D., Wittemann, J.K., and Ostenberg, P.V. The first dental visit for children from low socioeconomic families. *Journal of Dentistry for Children* 1974; *41*:376–81.

Heitkemper, T., Layne, C., and Sullivan, D.M. Brief treatment of children's dental pain and anxiety. *Perceptual and Motor Skills* 1993; *76*:192–94.

Hilgard, E.R. A neodissociation interpretation of pain reduction in hypnosis. *Psychological Review* 1973; *80*:396–411.

Hirschman, R., Young, D., and Nelson, C. Psychologically based techniques for stress reduction. In B.D. Ingersoll and W.R. McCutcheon (Eds.), *Clinical research in behavioral dentistry: proceedings of the second national conference on behavioral dentistry.* Morgantown, West Virginia, West Virginia University, 1979.

Hirschman, R. Physiological feedback and stress reduction. In B. Ingersoll (chair), Behavioral approaches to dental fear, pain and stress. Symposium presented at the meeting of Society of Behavioral Medicine, New York, 1980.

Hittelman, E. Presenting the obvious: dentists treat patients not teeth. *New York Journal of Dentistry* 1983; *53*(3):123–24.

Hodgson, R. and Rachman, S. Desynchrony measures of fear. *Behaviour Research and Therapy* 1974; *12*:319–26.

Hoffman, J.W., Benson, H., Arns, P.A., Stainbrook, G.L., Landsberg, G.L., Young, J.B., and Gill, A. Reduced sympathetic nervous system responsivity associated with the relaxation response. *Science* 1981; *215*:190–92.

Hogue, D., Ternisky, M., and Iranpour, B. The responses to nitrous oxide analgesia in children. *Journal of Dentistry for Children* 1971; *38*:129–33.

Hollister, L.E. *Clinical use of psychotherapeutic drugs.* Springfield, Ill.: Charles C. Thomas, 1973.

Houston, B.K. Control over stress, locus of control and response to stress. *Journal of Personality and Social Psychology* 1972; *21*:249–55.

Huwitt, J.W. and Stricker, G. Child patient response to various dental procedures. *Journal of the American Dental Association* 1965; *70*:70–74.

IASP subcommittee on Taxonomy. Pain terms with definitions and notes on usage. *Pain* 1979; *6*(3):249–52.

Ireland, R.L. Introducing the child to dentistry. *Journal of the American Dental Association* 1943; *30*:280–86.

Jackson, E. Patients' perceptions of dentistry. In P. Weinstein (Ed.), *Advances in behavioral research in dentistry.* Seattle: University of Washington, 1978.

Jacobson, E. *Progressive relaxation.* Chicago: University of Chicago Press, 1938.

Janis, I.L. *Psychological stress*. New York: Academic Press Inc., 1974, p. 284.

Jenks, L. How the dentist's behavior can influence the child's behavior. *Journal of Dentistry for Children* 1964; *31*:358–66.

Johnson, J.E., Levanthal, H., and Dabbs, J.M., Jr. Contribution of emotional and instrumental response processes in adaption to surgery. *Journal of Personality and Social Psychology* 1971; *20*:55–64.

Johnson, R. and Baldwin, D.C. Relationship of maternal anxiety to behavior of young children undergoing dental extractions. *Journal of Dental Research* 1968; *47*:801–05.

Johnson, R. and Baldwin, D.C. Maternal anxiety and child behavior. *Journal of Dentistry for Children* 1969; *36*:87–92.

Jones, M.C. The case of Peter. *Pedagogical Seminary* 1924; *31*:308–15.

Kanfer, F.H. and Goldfoot, D.A. Self-control and tolerance of noxious stimulation, *Psychological Reports* 1966; *18*:79–85.

Kardachi, B.J. and Clarke, N.G. The use of biofeedback to control bruxism. *Journal of Periodontology* 1977; *48*:639–42.

Kaufman, E., Weinstein, P., and Milgrom, P. Difficulties in achieving local anesthesia: a review. *Journal of the American Dental Association* 1984; *108*:205–08.

Kaufman, E., Hargreaves, K.M., and Dionne, R.A. Comparison of oral triazolam and nitrous oxide with placebo and intravenous diazepam for outpatient premedication. *Oral Surgery, Oral Medicine, Oral Pathology* 1993; *75*:156–64.

Kazdin, A.E. and Wilcoxon, L.A. Systematic desensitization and nonspecific treatment effects: A methodological evaluation. *Psychological Bulletin* 1976; *83*:729–58.

Kenney, E.B., Saxe, S.R., Lenox, J.A., Cooper, T.M., Caudill, I.S., Collins, A.R., and Kaplan, A. The relationship of manual dexterity and knowledge to performance of oral hygiene. *Journal of Periodontal Research* 1976; *11*(2):67–73.

Kiyak, H.A., Beach, B.H., Worthington, P., Taylor, T., Bolender, C., and Evans, E. The psychological impact of osseointergated dental implants.*International Journal of Maxillofacial Implants* 1990; *5*:61–69.

Kleber, C., Putt, M.S., and Muhler, J.C. Duration and pattern of toothbrushing in children using a gel or paste dentifrice. *Journal of the American Dental Association* 1981; *103*(5):723–26.

Kleinhauz, M., Eli, I., Baht, R., and Shamay, D. Correlates of success and failure in behavior therapy for dental fear. *Journal of Dental Research* 1992; *71*:1832–35.

Kleinknecht, R.A., Klepac, R.K., and Alexander, L.D. Origins and characteristics of fear of dentistry. *Journal of the American Dental Association* 1973; *86*:842–45.

Kleinknecht, R.A. and Bernstein, D.A. Assessment of dental fear. *Behavior Therapy* 1978; *9*:626–34.

Kleinknecht, R.A., McGlynn, F.D., Thorndike, R.M., and Harkavy, J. Factor analysis of the Dental Fear Survey with cross validation. *Journal of the American Dental Association* 1984; *108*:59–61.

Klepec, R.K. Successful treatment of avoidance of dentistry by desensitization or by increasing pain tolerance. *Journal of Behavioral Therapy and Experimental Psychology* 1975; *6*:307–12.

Klorman, R., Ratner, J., Arata, C.L., King, J.B., Jr., and Sveen, O.B. Predicting the child's uncooperativeness in dental treatment from maternal traits, state and dental anxiety. *Journal of Dentistry for Children* 1978; *45*:62–67.

Klorman, R., Michael, R., Hilpert, P.L., and Sveen, O.B. A further assessment of predictors of the child's behavior in dental treatment. *Journal of Dental Research* 1979; *58*:2338–43.

Korsch, B. and Aley, E. Pediatric interviewing techniques. *Current Problems in Pediatrics* 1973; *3*:1–42.

Kraper, D.C. Some behavioral topics related to dentistry, speech and audiology. Presented at Conference of Joint Committee for Dentistry and Speech Pathology–Audiology, Ann Arbor, Michigan, March 6, 1970.

Kress, G.C., Jr. Patient satisfaction with dental care. *Dental Clinics of North America* 1988; *Oct 32*(4):791–802.

Kroeger, R.F. *Managing the apprehensive dental patient.* Cincinnati: Heritage Communications, 1987.

Kuno, Y. *Human perspiration.* Springfield, IL: Thomas, 1956.

Kuster, C.G., and Rakes, G. Frequency of inadequate local anesthetic in child patients. *Journal of Paediatric Dentistry* 1987; *3*:7–9.

Langa, H. *Relative analgesia in dental practice.* Philadelphia: Saunders, 1968.

Langer, E.G., Janis, L.L., and Wolfer, J.A. Reduction of psychological stress in surgical patients. *Journal of Experimental and Social Psychology* 1975; *11*:155–65.

Laufer, D., Chosack, A., and Rosenzweig, K.A. Explanation as a means of reducing fear of dental procedures in children. *Alpha Omegan* 1964; *57*:130–33.

Lautch, H. Dental phobia. *British Journal of Psychiatry* 1971; *119*:151–58.

Lazarus, R.S. Some principles of psychological stress and their relation to dentistry. *Journal of Dental Research* 1966; *45*:1620–26.

Lazarus, R.S. The stress and coping paradigm. In C. Eisdorfer, D. Cohen, A. Kleinman, and P. Maxim (Eds.), *Models for clinical psychopathology*. Jamaica, New York: Spectrum Publications, 1981.

Lechner, V. and Wright, G.Z. Non-pharmacotherapeutic approaches to behavior management of the child patient. In G.Z. Wright (Ed.), *Behavior management in dentistry for children*. Philadelphia: W.B. Saunders, 1975.

Levitas, T.C. Hand over mouth exercise. *Journal of Dentistry for Children* 1974; *19*:178–82.

Lewis, T.M. and Law, D.B. Investigation of certain autonomic responses of children to specific dental stress. *Journal of the American Dental Association* 1958; *57*:769–77.

Lick, J. and Bootzin, R. Expectancy factors in the treatment of fear: methodological and theoretical issues. *Psychological Bulletin* 1975; *82*:917–31.

Liddell, A., DiFazio, L., Blackwood, J., and Ackerman, C. Long-term follow-up of treated dental phobics. *Behaviour Research and Therapy* 1994; *32*:605–10.

Litt, M.D., Nye, C., and Shafer, D. Coping with oral surgery by self-efficacy enhancement and perceptions of control. *Journal of Dental Research* 1993; *72*:1237–43.

Liu, H.H., Milgrom, P., and Fiset, L. Effect of a beta-adrenergic blocking agent on dental anxiety. *Journal of Dental Research* 1991; *70*:1306–08.

Locker D, Liddell A, and Burman D. Dental fear and anxiety in an older adult population. *Community Dentistry and Oral Epidemiology* 1991; *19*:120–24.

Logan, H.L., Baron, R.S., Keeley, K., Law, A., and Stein, S. Desired and felt control as mediators of stress in a dental setting. *Health Psychology* 1991; *10*:352–59.

Longley, A.J., Fiset, L., Getz, T., Van Arsdel, P.P., and Weinstein, P. Fear can mimic latex allergy in patients with dental phobia. *General Dentistry* 1994; 42:236–41.

Longo, D.J. A psychophysiological comparison of three relaxation techniques and some implications for testing cardiovascular syndromes. *Social and Behavioral Medicine Abstracts*, 1984; #A11, 10.

Macgreggor, I.D. and Rugg-Gunn, A.J. Survey of toothbrushing duration in 85 uninstructed English school children. *Community Dentistry and Oral Epidemiology* 1979; 7:297–98.

Machen, J.B. and Johnson, R. Desensitization, model learning, and the dental behavior of children. *Journal of Dental Research* 1974; 53:83–87.

Marks, I. *Fears and Phobias*. New York: Academic Press, 1969.

Martin, R.B., Shaw, M.A., and Taylor, P.P. The influence of prior surgical experience on the child's behavior at the initial dental visit. *Journal of Dentistry for Children* 1977; 44:443–47.

Mason, R.C., Clark, G., Reeves, R.B., and Wagner, S.B. Acceptance and healing. *Journal of Religion and Health* 1969; 8:123–42.

Mathews, A. Fear-reduction research and clinical phobia. *Psychological Bulletin* 1978; 85:390–404.

Mayo, R.W. Child management in the dental office. *Journal of Dentistry for Children* 1945; 12:48–49.

McGrath, P.A. Pain in children: Nature, assessment and treatment. New York: Guilford, 1990.

Melamed, B.G., Yurcheson, R., Fleece, E.L., Hutcherson, S., and Hawes, R. Effects of film modeling on the reduction of anxiety-related behaviors in individuals varying in level of previous experience in the stress situation. *Journal of Consulting and Clinical Psychology* 1978; 46:1357–67.

Melamed, S.F. *Handbook of local anesthesia*. St Louis: Mosby, 1990.

Mellor, A.C. Dental anxiety and attendance in the north-west of England. *Journal of Dentistry* 1992; 20:207–10.

Melzack, R., Weisz, A.Z., and Sprague, L.T. Strategies for controlling pain: Contributions of auditory stimulation and suggestion. *Experimental Neurology* 1963; 8:239–47.

Melzack, R. *The puzzle of pain*, New York: Basic Books, 1973.

Melzack, R., Guit, E.S., and Gonshor, A. Relief of dental pain by ice massage of the hand. *Canadian Medical Association Journal* 1980; 122:189–91.

Milgrom, P., Weinstein, P., and Kaufman, E. Student difficulties in achieving local anesthesia. *Journal of Dental Education* 1984; 48(3):168–70.

Milgrom, P., Fiset, L., Melnick, S., and Weinstein, P. The prevalence and practice management consequences of dental fear in a major US city. *Journal of the American Dental Association* 1988; 116:641–47.

Milgrom, P., Weinstein, P., Melnick, S., Beach, B., and Spadafora, A. Health risk assessment and oral hygiene instruction in dental practice. *Journal of Public Health Dentistry* 1989; 49(1):24–31.

Milgrom, P., Kleinknecht, R.A., Elliott, J., Liu, H.H., and Teo, C.S. A cross cultural cross validation of the Dental Fear Survey in South East Asia. *Behaviour Research and Therapy* 1990; 28:227–33.

Milgrom, P., Fiset, L., and Weinstein, P. Nonalcohol-based chlorhexidine dental rinse. *The Annals of Pharmacotherapy* 1992; 26:842.

Milgrom, P., Vignehsa, H., and Weinstein, P. Adolescent dental fear and control: Prevalence and theoretical implications. *Behaviour Research and Therapy* 1992; 30:367–73.

Milgrom, P. and Weinstein, P. Dental fears in general practice: New guidelines for assessment and treatment. *International Dental Journal* 1993; 43:288–93.

Milgrom, P., Weinstein, P., Roy-Byrne, P., and Tay, K.M. Dental fear treatment outcomes for substance use disorder patients. *Special Care in Dentistry* 1993; 13:1–4.

Milgrom, P., Weinstein, P., Fiset, L., and Beirne, O.R. The anxiolytic effects of intravenous sedation using midazolam alone in multiple drug techniques. *Journal of Oral and Maxillofacial Surgery* 1994; 52:219–24.

Milgrom, P., Mancl, L., King, B., and Weinstein, P. Origins of childhood dental fear: Rachman's theory of fear acquisition applied to a specific fear. *Behaviour Research and Therapy*, in press.

Milgrom, P., Mancl, L., King, B., Weinstein, P., Jeffcott, E., and Wells, N. An explanatory model of the dental care utilization of low-income children. *Medical Care*, in press.

Milgrom, P., Quarnstrom, F.C., and Longley, A. The efficacy and memory effects of oral triazolam premedication in highly anxious dental patients. *Anesthesia Progress*, in press.

Milgrom, P., Weinstein, P., Golletz, D., Leroux, B., and Domoto, P. The management of pain in school-aged children by dentists in private and public clinic practice. *Journal of Pediatric Dentistry*, in press.

Miller, N. and Dollard, J. *Personality and Psychotherapy*. New York: McGraw-Hill, 1950.

Miller, N.E. Learning of visceral and glandular response. *Science* 1969; *103*:434–45.

Miller, S.M. Controllability and human stress: Method, evidence and theory. *Behavioral Research and Therapy* 1979; *17*:287–304.

Molin, C. and Seeman, K. Disproportionate dental anxiety: clinical and nosological considerations. *Acta Odontologica Scandinavia* 1979; *28*:197–212.

Moore, P.A. and Dunsky, J.L. Bupivacaine anesthesia—A clinical trial for endodontic therapy. *Oral Surgery* 1984; *55*(2):176–79.

Moore, R. and Brodsguard, I. Group therapy compared with individual desensitization for dental anxiety. *Community Dentistry and Oral Epidemiology* 1994; *22*:258–62.

Moretti, R.J., Curtiss, G., and Hoerman, K.C. Dentist non-verbal communication skills, patient anxiety and patient treatment satisfaction. *Journal of Dental Research* 1982; *61*:264.

Muris, P., De Jongh, A., Van Zuuren, F.J., Ter Horst, G. Coping style, anxiety, cognitions, and cognitive control in dental phobia. *Personality and Individual Differences* 1994; *17*:143–45.

Mussellman, R. and McClure, D. In G.Z. Wright (Ed.), *Behavioral management in dentistry for children*. Philadelphia: Saunders, 1975.

Musselman, R.J. Considerations in behavior management of the pediatric patient. *Pediatric Clinics of North America* 1991; *38*:1309–24.

Nash, D.A., Ingersoll, B.D., and Gamber, C. Contingent audiotaped reinforcement with pediatric dental patients. *Journal of Dental Research* 1984; *63*:272.

Nathan, J. Assessment of anxious pedodontic patients to nitrous oxide. *Journal of Dental Research* 1982; *61*:224.

Nathan, J.E. Nitrous oxide and the management of fear and anxiety in children. In R. Moretti and W.A. Ayer (Eds.), *The president's conference of the dentist-patient relationship and the management of fear, anxiety and pain*, Chicago, Ill.: American Dental Association, 1983.

Neiburger, E.J. Child response to suggestion. *Journal of Dentistry for Children* 1978; *45*:396–402.

Neidle, E.A. and Yagiela, J.A. *Pharmacology and therapeutics for dentistry*, (3rd ed.). St. Louis: Mosby, 1989.

Neverlien, P.O. Dental fear and locus of control: a pilot study. *Community Dentistry and Oral Epidemiology* 1988; *16*(2):127.

Neverlien, P.O. Normative data for Corah's Dental Anxiety Scale (DAS) for the Norwegian adult population. *Community Dentistry and Oral Epidemiology* 1990; *18*:162.

Nikias, M. Compliance with preventive oral home care regimens. *Journal of Dental Research* 1980; *59*:2216–25.

Nippert, R.P. and Meier, T. Die Angst vor dem Zaharzt-Ergebnisse einer Erwachsenenbefragung. *Deutsche Zahnarztl Zeilschrift* 1987; *42*:939–43.

Oliver, C. and Hirschman, R. Voluntary heart rate control and perceived affects. *Journal of Dental Research* 1982; *61*:8–10.

Ollendick, T.H. and King, N.J. Origins of childhood fears: An evaluation of Rachman's theory of fear acquisition. *Behaviour Research and Therapy* 1991; *29*:117–23.

Öst, L.G. Individual response patterns and the effects of different behavioural methods in the treatment of phobias. In D. Magnusson and A. Ohman (Eds.). *Psychopathology*. New York: Academic Press, 1987.

Papermaster, A.A. A psychological study of the dental patient. *Northwest Dentistry* 1971; *50*:149–54.

Persson, G. General side-effects of local dental anesthesia. *Acta Odontologica Scandinavia* 1969; *27*(supplement):53.

Petersen, J.K. and Milgrom, P. *Pain relief in the oralfacial regions*. Copenhagen: Munksgaard, 1989.

Pollack, S. Pain control by suggestion. *Journal of Oral Medicine* 1966; *21*:89–95.

Quarnstrom, F.C., Milgrom, P., and Moore, P.A. Experience with triazolam in preschool children. *Anesthesia Pain Control in Dentistry* 1992; *1*:157–59.

Rachman, S. and Hodgson, R.I. Synchrony and disynchrony in fear and avoidance. *Behavioral Research and Therapy* 1974; *12*:311–18.

Rachman, S.J. *Fear and Courage,* 2nd ed, New York: Freeman & Co., 1990

Ramsay, D., Weinstein, P., Milgrom, P., and Getz, T. Problematic gagging: Principles of treatment. *Journal of the American Dental Association* 1987; *114*:178–83.

Rayman, M.S. Parent observation. *CDA Journal* 1987; *12*:20–24.

Rayman, M.S. From Seuss to Moss: Pediatric dental literature. *California Dental Association Journal* 1994; *22*:24–31.

Reiss, S. Pavlovian conditioning and human fear: an expectancy model. *Behavioral Therapy* 1980; *11*:300–96.

Richardson, S.S. and Kleinknecht, R.A. Expectancy effects on anxiety and self-generated cognitive strategies in high and low dental anxious females. Presented to Washington State Psychological Association Meeting, May, 1983.

Ripa, L. and Barenie, J.T. *Management of dental behavior in children.* Littleton, Mass.: PSC Publishers, 1979.

Robinson, H.B. Toothbrushing habits of 405 persons. *Journal of the American Dental Association* 1946; *33*:1112–17.

Roder, R.E., Law, D., and Lewis, T. Physiological responses of dentists to the presence of a parent in the operatory. *Journal of Dentistry for Children* 1961; *28*:263–70.

Rogers, C.R. *On becoming a person.* Boston: Houghton Mifflin, 1961.

Rose, L.F. and Kaye, D. (Eds.). *Internal medicine for dentistry.* St. Louis: Mosby Co., 1983.

Rosengarten, M. The behavior of the preschool child at the initial dental visit. *Journal of Dental Research* 1961; *40*:373.

Rotter, J.B. Generalized expectancies for internal versus external control of reinforcement. *Psychological Monographs* 1966; *80*(1):1–28.

Rouleau, J., Ladouceur, R., and Dufour, L. Pre-exposure to the first dental treatment. *Journal of Dental Research* 1981; *60*:30–34.

Roy-Bryne, P., Milgrom, P., Tay, K.-M., Weinstein, P., and Katon, W. Psychopathology and psychiatric diagnosis in subjects with dental phobia. *Journal of Anxiety Disorders* 1994; *8*:19–31.

Rugh, J. *Biofeedback in dentistry: research in clinical application.* Phoenix, Arizona: Semantodontics, 1977.

Sackett, D.L. and Haynes, R.B. *Compliance with therapeutic regimens.* Baltimore, Maryland: The Johns Hopkins University Press, 1976.

Sawtell, R.O., Simon, J.F., and Simeonsson, R.J. The effects of five preparatory methods upon child behavior during the first dental visit. *Journal of Dentistry for Children* 1974; 41:37–45.

Schacter, S. and Singer, J.E. Cognitive, social and psychological determinants of emotional state. *Psychological Review* 1962; 69:379–99.

Schmitt, F.E. and Wooldridge, P.J. Psychological preparation of surgical patients. *Nursing Research* 1973; 22:108–16.

Schuurs, A.H., and Hoogstraten, J. Appraisal of dental anxiety and fear questionnaires: a review. *Community Dentistry and Oral Epidemiology* 1993; 21:329–39.

Schwarz, E. Dental anxiety in young adult Danes under alternative dental care programs. *Scandinavian Journal of Dental Research* 1990; 98:442–50.

Scott, D.S. and Hirschman, R. Psychological aspects of dental anxiety in adults. *Journal of the American Dental Association* 1982; 104:27–31.

Scott, D.S., Hirschman, R., and Schroder, K. Historical antecedents of dental anxiety. *Journal of the American Dental Association* 1984; 108:42–45.

Seeman, K. and Molin, C. Psychopathology, feelings of confinement and helplessness in the dental chair, and the relationship to the dentist in patients with disproportionate dental anxiety (DDA). *ACTA Psychiatrica Scandinavica* 1976; 54:81–91.

Seeman, M. and Evans, J.W. Alienation and learning in a hospital setting. *American Social Review* 1962; 27:727–82.

Seligman, M.E.P., Maier, S.F., and Solomon, R.L. Unpredictable and uncontrollable aversive events. In F.R. Brush (Ed.), *Aversive conditioning and learning*. New York: Academic Press, 1971.

Seligman, M.E.P. *Helplessness: On depression, development and death.* San Francisco: W.C. Freeman, 1975.

Shannon, I.L. and Isbel, G.M. Stress in dental patients: effect of local anesthetic procedures. *Dental Digest* 1963; 69:459–61.

Shapiro, D.N. Reactions of children to oral surgery experience. *Journal of Dentistry for Children* 1967; 34:97–99.

Shaw, D.W. and Thoresen, C.E. Effects of modeling and desensitization in reducing dental phobia. *Journal of Counseling Psychology* 1974; 21:415–20.

Shaw, E.G. and Routh, D.K. Effect of mothers presence on children's reaction to aversive procedures. *Journal of Pediatric Psychology* 1982; 7:33–42.

Sheehan, D.V., Ballenger, J., and Jacobsen, G. The treatment of endogenous anxiety with phobic, hysterical and hypochondriacal symptoms. *Archives of General Psychiatry* 1980; 37:51–59.

Sheehan, D.V. Panic attacks and phobias. *New England Journal of Medicine* 1982; 308:156–58.

Shoben, E.M. and Borland, L. An empirical study of the etiology of dental fears. *Journal of Clinical Psychology* 1954; 10:171–174.

Smith, T., Weinstein, P., Milgrom, P., and Getz, T. An evaluation of an institution-based dental fears clinic. *Journal of Dental Research* 1984; 63:272.

Solberg, W.K. and Rugh, J.D. The use of bio-feedback devices in the treatment of bruxism. *Journal of the Southern California State Dental Association* 1972; 40:852–53.

Sorenson, H.W. and Roth, G.I. A case for nitrous oxide-oxygen inhalation sedation: aid in the elimination of the child's fear of the needle. *Dental Clinics of North America* 1973; 17:769–81.

Sosa, R., Kennell, J., Klaus, M., Robertson, S., and Urrutia, J. The effect of a supportive comparison on perinatal problems, length of labor, and mother-infant interaction. *New England Journal of Medicine* 1980; 303:597–600.

Spreads, C. *Breathing—the ABC's.* New York: Harper and Row, 1978.

Starkey, P.E. Training office personnel to manage children. In G.Z. Wright (Ed.), *Behavior management in dentistry for children.* Philadelphia: W.B. Saunders, 1975.

Steblay, N.M. and Blaman, A.L. Reduction of fear during dental treatment through reattribution techniques. *Journal of the American Dental Association* 1982; 105:1006–09.

Sternbach, R.A. *Pain: psychophysiological analysis.* New York: Academic Press, 1968.

Stouthard, M.E.A. and Hoogstraten, J. Prevalence of dental anxiety in the Netherlands. *Community Denistry andt Oral Epidemiology* 1990; 18:139–42.

Svensson, P. and Petersen, J.K. Anesthetic effect of EMLA occluded with Orahesive Oral Bandages on oral mucosa. A placebo-controlled study. *Anesthesia Progress* 1992; 39:79–82.

Svensson, P., Bjerring, P., Arendt-Nielsen, L., and Kaaber, S. Hypoalgesic effect of EMLA and lidocaine gel applied on human oral mucosa: quantitative evaluation by sensory pain thresholds to argon laser stimulation. *Anesthesia Progress* 1993 Jan.–Feb.; *39(1–2)*:4–8.

Swoope, C. Predicting denture success. *Journal of Prosthetic Dentistry* 1973; *30*:860–65.

Szasz, T.J. and Hollender, M.H. A contribution to the philosophy of medicine—the basic models of the doctor-patient relationship. *Archives of Internal Medicine* 1956; *97*:585–92.

Teo, C.S., Foong, W., Lui, H.H., Vignehsa, H., Elliott, J., and Milgrom, P. Prevalence of dental fear in young adult Singaporeans. *International Dental Journal* 1990; *40(1)*:37–42.

ter Horst G. and deWit, CA. Review of behavioural research in dentistry 1987–1992: Dental anxiety, dentist-patient relationship, compliance and dental attendance. *International Dental Journal* 1993; *43*:265–78.

Thompson, K.F. Hypnosis in dental practice: clinical views. In M. Weisenberg (Ed.), *The Control of Pain*. New York: Psychological Dimensions, 1977.

Thompson, S.C. Will it hurt less if I can control it? Complex answer to a simple question. *Psychological Bulletin* 1981; *90*:89–101.

Valins, S. Cognitive effects of false heart rate feedback. *Journal of Personality and Social Psychology* 1966; *6*:400–08.

Valins, S. and Ray, A.A. Effects of Cognitive desensitization of avoidance behavior. *Journal of Personality and Social Psychology* 1967; *7*:345–50.

Venham, L.L. The effect of the parent's presence on the anxiety and behavior of children receiving dental treatment. Unpublished dissertation, Ohio State University, 1971.

Venham, L.L. T.V. helps young patients relax. *Dentistry Survey* 1977; *53*:98.

Venham, L.L., Murray, P., and Gaulin-Kremer, E. Child-rearing variables affecting the preschool child's response to dental stress. *Journal of Dental Research* 1979; *58*:2–45.

Vervoorn, J.M., Duinkerke, A.S.H., and Van de Poel, A.C.M. Angst voor de tandarts bij tandelozen. *Nederlands Tijdschrift voor Tandheelkunde* 1989; *96*:326–28.

Weinberger, D.A., Schwartx, G.E., and Davidson, R.J. Low-anxious, high-anxious and repressive coping styles: Psychometric patterns and behavioral and physiological responses to stress. *Journal of Abnormal Psychology* 1979; *88*:369–80.

Weiner, A.A. and Sheehan, D.V. Etiology of dental anxiety: Psychological trauma or CNS chemical imbalance? *General Dentistry* 1990; *38*:39–43.

Weinstein, P., Smith, T.A., and Packer, M.A. Method for evaluating patient anxiety and the interpersonal effectiveness of dental personnel: An exploratory study. *Journal of Dental Research* 1972; *50*:1324–26.

Weinstein, P., Smith, T.A., and Bartlett, R. A study of the dental student-patient relationship. *Journal of Dental Research* 1973; *52*:1287–92.

Weinstein, P., Milgrom, P., Ratener, P., Read, W., and Morrison, K. Dentist's perception of the patients: Relationship to quality of care. *Journal of Public Health Dentistry* 1978; *38*:10–21.

Weinstein, P., Domoto, P., Getz, T., and Enger, R. Reliability and validity of a measure of confidence in child management. *Journal of Dental Research* 1979; *58*(Special Issue A):408.

Weinstein, P., Domoto, P.K., and Getz, T. Difficult children: the practical experience of 145 private practitioners. *Pediatric Dentistry* 1981; *3*:303–05.

Weinstein, P., Domoto, P.K., Getz, T., and Enger, R. Reliability and validity of a measure of confidence in child management. *Pediatric Dentistry* 1981; *2*:7–9.

Weinstein, P., Getz, T., Ratener, P., and Domoto, P. The effects of dentists' behaviors on fear-related behaviors in children. *Journal of the American Dental Association* 1982; *104*:32–38.

Weinstein, P., Getz, T., Ratener, P., and Domoto, P. Behavior of dental assistants managing young children in the operatory. *Pediatric Dentistry* 1983; *5*:115–20.

Weinstein, P., Fiset, L., and Lancaster, B.L. Long-term assessment of a behavioral approach in plaque control using a multiple baseline design: the need for relapse research. *Patient Counseling and Health Education* 1984; *5*:135–40.

Weinstein, P., Getz, T., and Milgrom, P. *Oral self-care: strategies for preventive dentistry*, Reston, Virginia: Reston Publishing Co., Inc. 1985.

Weinstein, P., Milgrom, P., Kaufman, K., Fiset, L., and Ramsay, D. Efficacy of local anesthesia: Patient perceptions of failure to achieve optimal anesthesia. *General Dentistry* 1985; 33(3):218–20.

Weinstein, P., Domoto, P.K., and Holleman, E. The use of nitrous oxide in the treatment of children: results of a controlled study. *Journal of the American Dental Association* 1986; 112:325–31.

Weinstein, P., Milgrom, P., and Ramsay, D.S. Treating dental fears using nitrous oxide oxygen inhalation and system desensitization. *General Dentistry* 1988; 36:322–26.

Weinstein, P. and Nathan, J.E. The challenge of fearful and phobic children. *Dental Clinics of North America* 1988; 32:667–92.

Weinstein, P., Milgrom, P, Melnick, S., Beach, B., and Spadafora, A. How effective is oral hygiene instruction? Results after six and 24 weeks. *Journal of Public Health Dentistry* 1989; 49(1):32–38.

Weinstein, P., Getz, T., and Milgrom, P. *Oral Self Care: Strategies for Preventive Dentistry* (3rd ed.). Seattle: University of Washington Continuing Dental Education, 1991.

Weisenberg, M., Kreindler, M.L., Schachat, R., and Werboff, J. Interpreting palmar sweat prints: Not-so-simple measure. *Journal of Psychosomatic Research* 1976; 20:1–6.

Weisenberg, M. Cultural and racial reactions to pain. In M. Weisenberg (Ed.), *The control of pain*. New York: Psychological Dimension, 1977a.

Weisenberg, M. Pain and pain control. *Psychological Bulletin* 1977b; 84:1008–44.

Williams, J.A., Hurst, M.K., and Stokes, T.F. Peer observation in decreasing uncooperative behavior in young dental patients. *Behavior Modification* 1983; 7:225–42.

Winkler, S. Psychological aspects of treating complete denture patients: their relation to prosthodontic success. *Journal of Geriatric Psychiatry and Neurology* 1989; 2:48–51.

Wolpe, J. *Psychotherapy by reciprocal inhibition*. Stanford, CA: Stanford University Press, 1958.

Wright, F.A.C. Relationship of children's anxiety to the potential dental health behavior. *Community Dentistry and Oral Epidemiology* 1980; 8:189–94.

Wright, G.Z. and Alpern, G.D. Variables in fluencing children's cooperative behavior at the first dental visit. *Journal of Dentistry for Children* 1971; 38:60–64.

Wright, G.Z. *Behavior management in dentistry for children.* Philadelphia: Saunders, 1975.

Wright, G.Z., Alpern, G.D., and Leake, J.L. The modifiability of maternal anxiety as it relates to children's cooperative dental behavior. *Journal of Dentistry for Children* 1973; 40:265–71.

Wright, G.Z. and McAulay, D.J. Current premedicating trends in pedodontics. *Journal of Dentistry for Children* 1973; 55:185–87.

Wurster, C.A., Weinstein, P., and Cohen, A.J. Communication patterns in pedodontics. *Perceptual and Motor Skills* 1979; 48:159–66.

Yates, A.J. *Theory and practice in behavior therapy.* New York: John Wiley and Sons, 1970.

Index